D0206981

CHANGE
THE WAY
YOU GO TO THE
DENTIST

CHANGE THE WAY YOU GO TO THE DENTIST

MELVIN BENSON JR., DDS, FAGD

Advantage®

Copyright © 2019 by Melvin Benson, Jr.

All rights reserved. No part of this book may be used or reproduced in any manner whatsoever without prior written consent of the author, except as provided by the United States of America copyright law.

Published by Advantage, Charleston, South Carolina.
Member of Advantage Media Group.

ADVANTAGE is a registered trademark, and the Advantage colophon is a trademark of Advantage Media Group, Inc.

Printed in the United States of America.

10 9 8 7 6 5 4 3 2 1

ISBN: 978-1-59932-979-6
LCCN: 2018939830

Cover design by Melanie Cloth.
Layout design by Carly Blake.

This publication is designed to provide accurate and authoritative information in regard to the subject matter covered. It is sold with the understanding that the publisher is not engaged in rendering legal, accounting, or other professional services. If legal advice or other expert assistance is required, the services of a competent professional person should be sought.

Advantage Media Group is proud to be a part of the Tree Neutral® program. Tree Neutral offsets the number of trees consumed in the production and printing of this book by taking proactive steps such as planting trees in direct proportion to the number of trees used to print books. To learn more about Tree Neutral, please visit www.treeneutral.com.

Advantage Media Group is a publisher of business, self-improvement, and professional development books and online learning. We help entrepreneurs, business leaders, and professionals share their Stories, Passion, and Knowledge to help others Learn & Grow. Do you have a manuscript or book idea that you would like us to consider for publishing? Please visit advantagefamily.com or call 1.866.775.1696.

To my wife, Jenny, who without her love and support this dream would not be a reality. To my children, Rachel and Connor, who have had to share their time with dad for those who have needed help. And to my team at Integrated Dental who believe in our mission to truly change the way you go to the dentist.

Table of Contents

Part One: A Category of One

INTRODUCTION 3

CHAPTER 1 21
The Patient Centered Philosophy

CHAPTER 2 31
What is an Unhealthy Smile Costing You?

CHAPTER 3 41
Unleashing Human Potential

CHAPTER 4 51
Best Team in Town

CHAPTER 5 59
Steward of Your Smile

CHAPTER 6 73
Freedom Day USA: A Day of Free Dentistry

CHAPTER 7 81
Begin with the End in Mind

Part Two: Your Mouth at Every Age

CHAPTER 8 89
Childhood

CHAPTER 9 99
Pre-Teens and Teenagers

CHAPTER 10 109
Ages 20–39

CHAPTER 11 125
Ages 40–59

CHAPTER 12 137
Ages 60+

CONCLUSION 147

Part One

A Category of One

Introduction

President Andrew Jackson said, "I've got some big shoes to fill. This is my chance to do something. I have to seize the moment."

I guess anyone who grows up with a "Jr." after their name always feels they have something to live up to. It was that way with my dad—he was a dentist, and I knew in some way I wanted to follow in his footsteps, but I never felt it was any kind of pressure, or a competition. I was just like most kids who idolized their dad. In fact, my mother still loves to tell the story of how, when I could barely even walk, I would sit next to my dad and do lab work with him while wearing my own personal lab jacket that said "Jr. DDS."

I grew up in western Oklahoma. If a town had ten thousand people, that was a lot, and in our town, my dad was the "town dentist." He was one of your typical small-town heroes and therefore we couldn't go to a store, restaurant, or anywhere in town without running into someone who knew him. Now, that might bother some kids, but not me—I couldn't have been prouder of who I was. I loved being the son of one of the town's celebrities.

I knew, no matter what I did or where I went in life, I wanted to always bring that small town, southern charm to whatever business I went into. The exposure I had as a child in my dad's dental office paved the way for the development of how I approach dentistry and patients in my office today. I observed how to be more caring, more personable, and to really listen to people, which allows my patients to be at ease and connect with me, so I can get down to the root of their problem.

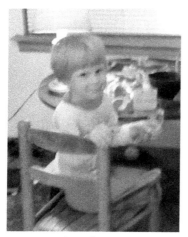
Dr. Benson doing "lab work" with his dad's dental equipment.

Growing up, I learned so much from watching my dad. He had a strong work ethic and was always striving to be the very best dentist he could be. He literally built his practice from the ground up, constructing his own building and growing his practice to become a pillar of the community. At that time, seeing him and how he worked, and how the community really loved him, I couldn't say that I wanted to be a dentist specifically, but I knew I wanted to be in the medical field and be the kind of practitioner he was.

Life went on like normal for a while until one day, when I was a junior in high school, my dad sustained a career-ending shoulder injury. Of course, he was devastated when he could no longer practice general dentistry. But given the kind of man he was, and his passion for helping people and for the field of dentistry, he did not let his injury stop him. He applied and was the first dentist from the Midwest to be accepted to the facial pain program at the University of Florida. He completed the fellowship program which focused on practicing diagnostic-based dentistry and dental medicine, which went beyond simple cavities and tooth restorations, and was not hindered by his disability. He had found his new calling within the field of dentistry, and he began helping patients with facial pain and issues that had not and could not be handled anywhere else. Instead of "drilling and filling," he was taking a whole-body approach, including health, history, and trauma, into account when diagnosing head and neck issues.

Around the same time, he had been named clinical director of The Parker Mahan Facial Pain Center, I was a junior in college and I was still trying to decide between the medical field and the dental field. I had decided to spend the week of spring break at the University of Florida and the pain center to research my options more thoroughly. My father and I spoke about the state of modern medicine, and where we both thought the medical field was going. I also had the opportunity to discuss the same subject with other dentists and even a few medical doctors. We were able to discuss the differences between the two fields, and I was coming to the quick conclusion that I could do more for my patients as a dentist rather than a medical doctor. These discussions were well before the Affordable Care Act, and yet, most, if not all the medical doctors I spoke with, were already complaining about their growing frustrations because they could not spend the necessary amount of time with each patient to provide the quality of care they had hoped to be able to when they first became physicians.

I knew, based on my memories and feelings from being a kid watching my dad with his patients, I wanted to be able to take my time and get to know my patients. I wanted to discover who they were, what problems they were experiencing, and how I could meet their needs and alleviate any issues they may be experiencing. I did not want a rushed, impersonal relationship with my patients. I did not want anyone, insurance, investor, or CEO, telling me who I could see, how long I could see them, or what procedures I was allowed or not allowed to complete as seen in several corporate dental facilities today.

This trip and these discussions led to my light bulb moment where I told myself I could have the best of both worlds. I could see that the practice of dentistry was already aligning more with traditional medicine, where the days of just "drilling and filling" were gone. The field of dentistry was growing into oral medicine and people were becoming more aware of the critical role good oral health plays into their overall health. I knew that I could combine the artistry of dentistry, the personal connection of being a hometown dentist, and still be a practitioner of medicine with the way dentistry was evolving into the practice of oral medicine. After talking with my dad and the other doctors, I realized that I wanted to be a dentist because I knew that was the field in which I could make the most positive impact on people's lives.

I applied was accepted to The University of Oklahoma School of Dentistry. My wife, Jenny, and I were married in June 2002 and after we returned from our honeymoon (in Disney World) I started dental school in July. Our daughter Rachel was born my junior year. My son Connor came along not long after I had purchased my first practice. My entire family has always been incredibly supportive and we share the goal of changing the way people view going to the dentist and the goal to change the lives of those in our community, not only through dentistry, but through community involvement. I graduated from OU in June 2006 and I hit the ground running in my dental career!

Integrated Dental

As I said before, I wanted to combine artistry of dentistry, the personal connection of being a hometown dentist, and still be a practitioner of medicine with the way dentistry was evolving into the practice of oral medicine. Interestingly enough, the road to my current practice did not start out meeting those expectations. When I first graduated from dental school, I went to work for one of those large, corporate dental offices for about nine months. As you might imagine, it was exactly the opposite of what I wanted out of dentistry, both personally and professionally. It was a painfully impersonal approach to patient interaction. Their philosophy was "treat as many patients as you can—get them in, complete treatment, maximize their insurance and bill them, and get them out the door as fast as possible." All they cared about was the numbers and how billable you could be. This approach was not for me at all, and looking back, it's hard to believe I even lasted nine months.

To facilitate my exit from corporate dentistry, I purchased a small practice in Oklahoma City. To show precisely how small the world truly is, the dental practice I purchased was my wife's family dentist, who was ready to sell and retire. While this professional experience was a little closer to my expectations of how I wanted to practice dentistry, something still wasn't right. We were close to our families, my team at the office was amazing, and just like family, the patients were wonderful and appreciative. The location was perfect—but still, something didn't fit. I continued to practice out of this office for five years, and in that time, I had my "ah-ha" moment and realized what was missing. Living and practicing in a large metropolitan area was not for me. I could not have the impact on the community in a place as big and disconnected as Oklahoma City.

Call it divine intervention, call it fate, call it luck, but a dentist approached me about purchasing my practice. This dentist was from Evergreen, Colorado. During the negotiations, I mentioned to him that since graduating dental school, I was licensed in both Oklahoma and Colorado, but had been unable to find a practice location in Colorado. He mentioned that I should look in northern Colorado, near the front range, and so I did. Within three months, I had found a practice. My wife and I visited Greeley and knew that was where we should be, so we signed the contracts in the Denver International Airport, and forty-five days later, had a U-Haul packed and we were on the way!

My wife and I fell in love with everything in Greeley. The practice I purchased was very small and the town itself only had about one hundred thousand people, but it felt like the small town I grew up in. I have now been living and practicing in Greeley for over six years, and I know I am finally in the place I want to be in, a place I can call home.

When deciding on a name for the practice, I finally chose Integrated Dental for many reasons. First, I wanted to integrate the whole health model of your healthy lifestyle begins with a healthy mouth. I also wanted to integrate the medicine and facial pain aspect into my dentistry. I wanted to integrate all facets of dentistry and only refer out rare and complicated cases. And finally, I wanted to integrate the goals and values—of changing the way you go to the dentist and changing the lives of those around me—to my team and my patients.

In Greeley, I am able to have the impact in the community that I've always wanted. My family, my team, and I are very active in the community, not just with patient care but in teaming up with the local food bank, community events, and our annual Freedom Day USA event. People know me, they know my brand and what I stand for. I can't walk into King Soopers or the Kum and Go without running into at least one patient or someone saying, "Hey Dr. Benson!"

Integrated Dental Vs "Corporate Dentistry"

When I was growing up, my dad ran a very small, quaint practice. He only had three chairs and one hygienist, and he just went back and forth between his patients as time permitted. Today, our ability to complete x-rays, diagnosis, and complete procedures is

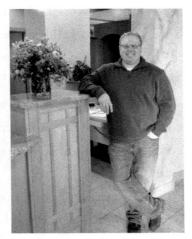

Dr. Benson on the first day of owning Integrated Dental Arts, December 31, 2012.

more advanced than even ten years ago. We have digital x-rays, which has the lowest radiation dose of all studies performed. We can make crowns chair-side in a single day during your appointment. And the latest technology, which I hope will soon become the standard of care in the field of dentistry, is a three-dimensional scan called cone beam (CBCT). With CBCT technology, we can see the head and neck in three dimensions, and we can treatment plan and complete delicate procedures such as dental implants and root canals more precisely.

Today, state-of-the-art dental technology is truly incredible. However, you cannot rely on the latest technology to define your practice. Technology can make a good dentist great. It can even sometimes make up for shortcomings in a not-so-good dentist. But the latest and greatest technology cannot help you connect with your patients. In fact, in some ways, it can even broaden the gaps between the dentist and the patient. In the midst of all technology, dental included, the human element and interaction has become increasingly more important.

During my brief stint in the corporate dental world, I learned a lot about how I did not want to practice dentistry. I continue to learn more about the corporate dental world today, even though I am a private practice owner. What the corporate dental chains fail to see when I worked for them or even now when one of their patients comes to our office for help, or when one of their management companies sends me a purchase offer, is what truly differentiates "us" from "them."

I am truly honored to own Integrated Dental. I am the sole owner of a dental practice that I am proud of. I not only own the

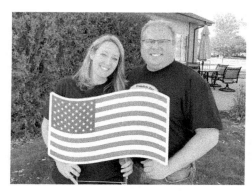

Dr. Benson and his wife Jenny on their Freedom Day USA event in 2018.

practice, but the building as well as a home in Greeley. I am not saying this to brag, I am simply pointing out that I love and support the town of Greeley, just as they support me. How can you truly understand your patients if you don't live and breathe the same community that they do? Yes, sometimes it is embarrassing when I run into a patient at King Soopers after I have been at the gym, but then again, they see that I am human too. In one of the large corporate dental offices, although owned by a licensed dentist(s), you may never see the owner/doctor. He may not even reside in the same state. If the owner doesn't understand the community that you are in, how can they understand who you are or your needs?

In my experience, I can say that the corporate dental chains do not care about the individual patient. I have seen this not only through my corporate experience, but also by listening to dozens of patients who have left one of the chains to come to Integrated

Dental. While I was an employee, I remember being told things such as, "Dr. Benson, we have this kid coming in today and there is $1,000 on their insurance, so we need to do as much work as possible because we don't know if he's coming back." Many of my patients who have previously been in a corporate office confess that it took years to work up the courage to return to the dentist because of their experience elsewhere.

That is another thing that separates us from them—in a corporate dental office there is no effort placed on patient retention, it is: "just do as much work as you can so you can maximize their bill and insurance on that first office visit." It was extremely bothersome how much my superiors focused on money. I've always been taught that if you do the right thing, then good things will come back to you. My personal goal is to help each patient get healthy while taking their needs, reservations, and means into account.

The truth is, in many ways, despite all we are doing to change the perceptions of the modern dentist, the corporate practices are giving general dentistry a bad name. In their world, it's all about the numbers. When you work there, you are given a production number— "this is the amount of revenue you need to produce each day." This number was to be reached by utilizing all means possible including maximizing treatment, allowing assistants to do work they were not qualified to do, and relying on technology that the staff may or may not have been properly trained on. That is not what I went into dentistry for; I want to do what the patient needs, not just what I can bill insurance for!

When I worked at one of those places, they would actually try and get me to do "over-treatment." Over-treatment could include x-rays that the patient was eligible for but did not need, larger fillings than were necessary, even crowns and extractions that were not necessary! Even today, while providing complimentary second opinions on treatment plans, I see a lot of over-treatment prescribed by the corporate dental offices. Especially in children. That was the last straw for me—you simply do not take advantage and over-treat kids! In our world, the patient is a person, not a number!

Who is Your Dentist?

With student loans on the rise and the cost of running a dental practice increasing, corporations are recruiting new graduates and retiring dentists by the truckload. With this new trend, it is now, more than ever, important to know "Who is Your Dentist?" What should you look for in your dentist? How can you tell if a dental practice is privately owned or a corporation?

- *What is your first impression?* When you call, does the person answering the phone address your reason for calling, or are they trying to sell you on a "special" they have running? Not that a special isn't good, because patients can often save money on diagnostic treatment such as exams and x-rays, but how low is too low? When you arrive for your appointment, what does the lobby look like? Have they updated their office in this decade? Do they have updated equipment, and do they use digital technology to reduce the amount of radiation exposure? These are observations and questions that are incredibly important as you choose your dentist.

- *Have you read any of the dental office reviews?* Before becoming a new patient, you should research your new dentist by not only reading the online reviews regarding the office but the reviews and biographies of the specific dentist that you are going to see. Many offices have multiple dentists, and you want to make sure you are seeing the dentist that is qualified to treat your condition. Corporate chains will often keep the name of the dental practices they purchase and therefore they will retain reviews of the practice of each particular practice. Why is this important? Although reviews, website names, and locations are retained, sometime the staff is not. Be aware of this—you may not be seeing the same doctor that you used to. As a patient, it is your right to ask, "Who owns the practice?" and "Does that doctor work here?" If they give you a name you have never heard of, then chances are they are owned by someone else, or even a corporation, and neither may even live in your town or state!

- **Is the office obsessed with money?** Do they present finances and payment options before you have even seen the doctor? In my corporate experience, my team had a "daily goal" that we were required to meet. Your dental issue that led you to make the appointment may not even be what this dental office currently wants to treat.

As we age, prevention is the key to longevity. Our teeth are no different. Good oral hygiene, regular cleanings, check-ups, and x-rays are a necessity. Do not be fooled by those who do not have your health or interests first.

A Different Patient Experience

As you might imagine, the emphasis on being "patient-centric" results in a very different patient experience. I realize many people still have a fear of the dentist. We are the "scary guys in white coats" that include bad memories from way back when you were children. I do not want to be that guy. One of the things I remember so clearly from my corporate experience is the distinct "smell of the doctor's office" everyone knows. If you walk into a dentist's office and smell that typical unappealing disinfectant scent and dental materials, it can bring back all those negative feelings about seeing the dentist from childhood. Smells can easily trigger emotions and memories. However, you won't smell anything like that when you walk through the doors of Integrated Dental.

I wanted my practice to smell like home, or look and feel like you just walked into the lobby of a fine hotel. When our patients walk through the doors, they'll immediately notice the room is filled with sunshine. Fresh flowers sit on our beverage bar and the light aroma of essential oils can be smelled throughout the office. Our front desk team will stand up, smile, and greet you by name. There is no annoying, sliding glass door and there's no barrier between our reception desk and the patient—there's just a countertop. Everything is open and transparent, literally; there is a glass door that patients can see through and into our clinical department.

I do not have a TV in my waiting room, because my philosophy is, you shouldn't be in my waiting room long enough to watch TV! That is another one of my pet peeves—I think your time is as valuable as my own. Your waiting time should always be minimal. Of course, we make you feel welcome and comfortable while you are waiting. We have coffee, juice, water, as well as books (mostly for kids) and magazines. We even have a comfort menu with amenities to make your visit to our office more pleasant. Some of our comfort menu items include headphones, paraffin hand dip, and blankets just to name a few.

The whole idea is to make our patients feel welcome and comfortable, like they are walking into someone's home. I want them to feel like they chose the right dentist and they are in good hands from the moment they step inside our front doors, particularly if they are coming with children. If we can eliminate that fear of the dentist when a child comes in for their first visit, we are setting him or her up for a lifetime of good oral health.

Children and Dental Phobia

When parents come in with young children, we take a very conservative approach. The first appointment is always what we call a "Happy Visit," where they sit in the dental chair, we brush their teeth a little, and we let them play with some dental equipment like the suction tool. I tell all parents that when I see kids, my primary job is to make them unafraid of the dentist. And I am going to do everything in my power to make sure they see me as their friend and helper, "Dr. Buddy," and not the monster in the white coat. The child's interests always come first. Sometimes that means I may have to refer them to a pedodontist for sedation if I think they need that. This way they go to sleep, they wake up, and they're done—no pain, no fear. Once I even had to send my own daughter to the pedodontist so she could relax!

We never force a child to have a procedure they are truly scared of. We will try some tricks of the trade, however. There's one called "tell, show, do" that many dentists use. We tell them what we're going to do, we then show them what we're going to do, and then we do it. But, even in doing so, if I feel the child is not ready for it, we certainly will never push them. Other than emergencies, of course, there is no real given age that a child is definitely ready for his or her first visit. Some kids are ready at two, some kids aren't ready till five or six, and that's really individually based on the child. It's all about making it fun, and making it personal. I tell the parents, "here are the habits we want you to get into," so when we do "tell, show, do," it's not just for the kids, it's also for the parents, because there's no dental handbook for parents, or at least there wasn't until the one you are reading!

We Are Not Just Treating Teeth— We Are Changing Lives

At Integrated Dental, I feel that we are not just doing dentistry, we are changing people's lives for the better. Yes, we are improving smiles, but cosmetics is not our main focus. Having a beautiful smile is great because it is the first thing people notice, but having a healthy smile that is functional will last you a lifetime. The ability to chew and function well into your seventies, eighties, or beyond, is a far more important than cosmetics. This is why I tell all my patients that we focus on health first, function second, and only after do we look at aesthetics. My first goal as a medical professional is to make sure you are healthy.

I am sure you have heard the old saying that "form follows function." Usually, if I get you to function well, looking good naturally follows. That's really where my passion resides—restoring patients' mouths and/or replacing missing teeth, or getting them back the ability to chew and smile confidently. I get so many patients who come in and say, "I can't chew a salad anymore," or "I can't bite into a steak." One of the most rewarding moments in my practice is when I can do a denture, or some other kind of restoration, and the patient calls me the next day and lets me know how I have changed his or her life. I had a patient recently call me and say, "Hey Doc, I was chewing jelly beans today—I haven't chewed jelly beans in years!"

I have a lot of patients who come in feeling very embarrassed by their smile, or the condition of their teeth. At Integrated Dental, we don't judge. I am probably the least judgmental person you will ever meet. It is important to understand that each person's life and genetic circumstances are different, and it is not important how the condition happened, it is only important that we are here to help each patient get healthy.

I find a way to let our patients know they have no reason to be shy or embarrassed, as there are so many reasons that teeth can deteriorate. My ultimate goal is to make every patient comfortable, to the point where he or she feels like they can tell me anything, so we can really get down to the root of the problem. I think that is my greatest strength as a healer. It's being empathetic and still managing to get the job done, and having the patient feel really good when they walk out.

This goes back to one of my very first experiences as a private practice owner. I had only owned my Oklahoma City practice a little over a year when I had a patient present to me wanting to fix her teeth because she had been abused. None of her teeth were savable. She was looking at having to do implants and a snap-on denture for both the upper and the lower arches. She did not have the funds for that kind of work, but I talked to the oral surgeon and said, "We've got to help this lady out."

We worked out a minimal price, did all the implants, made the full dentures, and when she snapped those dentures in and looked in the mirror, she broke out into tears—tears of joy of course, because she didn't think she could ever be whole again. We put her back together.

Within that same year, she got herself a job, and she found a boyfriend. We helped this patient turn her life around! She was one of my first patients, and I have helped countless others since then. I have an amazing sense of gratitude and realize how lucky I am to be in this field and that I have been given the ability to change the lives of so many people.

Giving Back

The amount of people we've been able to affect and the lives we've changed since moving to Colorado never ceases to amaze me. It is very humbling. Being here has given me the opportunity to do what I have always wanted to do, not only change the individual lives of my patients, but to give back to the community.

We do something called Freedom Day USA. It's a day where we provide free dental care to veterans and their spouses. Over the last six years, as a combined effort, we've given away over a $350,000 in free dentistry. This is not just having them come in for cleanings and simple fillings. These patients are getting full dental care. They're getting crowns, they're getting dentures, and they're getting full mouth restorations. These are people that served our country, and they deserve to see that they are appreciated, and that we can change their lives, because someone cares.

Changing the Way You Go to the Dentist

Changing lives is what dentistry has always been to me. It is about the people I can help and the lives I can change for the better. I know you can choose any dentist, but I hope you will come to understand who I am, and how I am different. My slogan is, "Changing the way you go to the dentist," and that is what I am committed to doing.

One of the biggest compliments I get—and barely a day goes by where I do not hear it—is when a patient says, "This is different than any other dental office I've ever been to." When I hear that, I know we are doing something right, because I don't want to be like everybody else. Everybody else is doing it "the old way"—what I like to call "tooth dentistry," where you treat one tooth and one problem. The patient comes in with a problem, you treat that tooth, and then the patient is gone. That is the old way of doing things, and unfortunately, the way they are still doing things in corporate dentistry. But here, not only do we treat you as an individual, we also recognize that we have to treat the entire system. This is how we are transforming dentistry into "oral medicine."

You have to treat the teeth, the jaw, the muscles—you have to treat the patients, and get to know them and their lifestyle. To me, that is the difference between a quality dentist and somebody that's just out for a paycheck. It is someone who is interested in you, in your life story, your overall health, your likes, dislikes, your hobbies and your families.

I want readers to walk away from this book and realize that while the tools may be the same, not every dentist is the same. At Integrated Dental, we want to get to know the patient before we get to know their problem. This way you will know from the very beginning that our focus is on you, and not just your tooth problem. When there is that personal touch, it can literally make a lifetime worth of difference, not only my patients, but for myself and my staff.

Chapter 1

THE PATIENT CENTERED PHILOSOPHY

Tell me if this sounds familiar: You open the door to a dental office and the first thing you notice is the harsh smell of disinfectant. There are a bunch of old, worn out chairs lining the walls—none of which are comfortably facing the television screen that's displaying static—and stacks of outdated lifestyle magazines are scattered on the scarce side tables. And at the furthest end of the room is a sliding glass window, scratched and smudged with fingerprints. Behind them sits an assistant who somehow doesn't see you standing at said window for at least two or three minutes after you've arrived.

At some point, our society to accept this kind of treatment as the norm; that we weren't people as much as we were penitents, come to beg for a moment of time with the almighty Doctor, and even if we'd scheduled an appointment, we were willing to wait for hours—

half our day, even—for what ultimately amounts to five minutes of attention.

This is not how it should be.

---

5 Reasons People Don't Like Doctor Visits

From the Huffington Post

1. The doctor doesn't listen
2. The long wait
3. The doctor doesn't care
4. The doctor makes too much money
5. My dog gets more respect

A large part of the dissatisfaction with dental visits is created by the environment and the doctor's non-patient-centric approach to delivering treatment. Most people's perception of a dental office, in other words, is that sliding glass window, the clipboard of medical questions, and the long wait until you're beckoned behind the door and into a treatment room. From the moment a patient steps in the front door, they're treated like a piece of paperwork because in the end, that's really all they're seen as.

The Patient Centered Practice Model

Our office couldn't be further from this dated, frustrating approach. For one, we don't even *have* a sliding glass window.

Words that Describe a Patient Centered Model

- Comfortable
- Relaxed
- Understood
- Important
- Satisfied
- Listened to
- Cared for
- Respected

The system we have created in our office is what's called the Patient Centered Model. The entire dental experience is crafted around putting you, the patient, first, with predetermined steps that include speed when speed is necessary, clear communication, and treatment that is well above the norm.

Creating a Five-Star Patient Experience

When you walk into our office, our focus is on getting you to where you need to be as fast as possible, streamlining paperwork so that there's ample time to spend with the doctor for your questions and procedure. To accomplish this, we extensively train our team on what both the patient and the doctor require so there are as few hiccups in the process as possible.

This attention to detail and process goes well beyond the evident. For instance:

- ***Answering the phone right away.*** This may seem obvious, but try calling your physician right now. If you're like most, your call was probably received by an automated answering service that made you pick a number, and then another number, and possibly even a third number, just so you can leave a message on an answering machine. This is not the case at our office. Our phones are answered quickly by a real person so that we can address your needs promptly.

- ***Flexible Schedule.*** We strive to keep flexibility in our schedule so that if the need occurs, we can see you quickly—if not the same day—at a time that's as convenient as possible. One of our mottos has always been "Emergencies Seen Same Day." We also have extended hours, including early morning and evening hours, so you can miss less time at work or school for your dental appointments.

- ***Clean Spaces.*** Every space associated with our office, from our parking area to the storage closet, is kept clean and in good condition. The sign for our office is easy to read from the street, so you know you're at the right place. The common areas and restrooms are clean and comfortable, and lightly scented so that they don't smell medical while at the same time, not overpoweringly fragrant. And there's no such thing as a worn or dirty surface in our office space. We make it a point to keep *all* glass surfaces clean, the paint fresh, and the furniture in good, clean condition.

- ***Reception Desk.*** Gone are the days of the non-responsive front desk person behind a tiny sliding glass window. Not only have we removed the window, but the front desk is also open and uncluttered, with a smiling patient coordinator that greets you the moment you walk up.

- **Patient Amenities**. Our waiting room is clean and tidy, with reading material for all ages and free wi-fi. We also offer our patients and their family members that may be accompanying them a fully stocked beverage bar including coffee, bottled water, and juice. Patients receiving treatment can request other items from our comfort menu to make their visit more enjoyable. Some of these items include a complimentary paraffin hand dip, essential oils, blankets, and headphones to listen to music or watch movies.

- **Treatment Rooms.** We understand that the fear factor for dental offices is real and pervasive in our society. When designing and outfitting our new dental space in our current building, we did not compromise or spare any expense on getting the best equipment to use to treat our patients. We have invested in state-of-the-art technology including the newest dental chairs and delivery systems, digital scans for some impressions, E4D Crowns in a Day, digital x-rays, and cone beam CT.

- **Inform Before We Perform.** Although this may seem obvious, we have had many new patients come to our office because their previous dentist did not completely inform them of all dental procedures available to them. Our philosophy has always been to inform the patient before we perform any procedure. This information would include treatment plan and procedure options (as there can be more than one option to fix a problem), possible side effects, guarantees and warranties, financial obligations and arrangements, and post procedure care.

Perception Is Everything

A story I've often heard attributed to Don Burr, founder of the former People Express Airlines, does an excellent job of pointing out the importance of attention to every detail.

Picture yourself the last time you had to fly somewhere. Imagine you had a pretty ideal experience this time around—you checked in early online, the line for security was minimal, and your gate was conveniently close to a cafe with clean, available tables. When they called your flight, you got onboard without a hitch, found a spot for your luggage right over your seat, and got into your seat without stepping over two other people or ticking off the other passengers around you.

Everything was going brilliantly until you sat down and unfolded the tray table and there, on the surface of the table, was a huge, crusty food stain. In that moment, you suddenly became convinced that the pilot was incompetent, the wings were held on with duct tape and the engine was one decrepit shiver from bursting into flame.

Perception is everything, and if we aren't paying attention to detail, then dentists can be rest assured that their clients *are*.

Everything about your visit, from the moment you arrive, should feel like a five-star experience.

A fair number of patient satisfaction surveys suggest that while patients may like their doctor, they are most dissatisfied with the treatment they received from supporting team members. This is why our focus is a complete 180 degrees from the typical medical office experience—we spend an enormous amount of energy and effort making sure that our team is always present and aware of our clients' needs. Our staff know—and agree—that their needs come second to the needs of our patients.

From the moment you walk in the door, your experience dictates your relationship with us. Creating the best first impression requires substantial energy and effort, but if the end result is that our clients feel more comfortable, less fearful, and more respected by our doctors and staff, then it's all worth it.

Category of One

What is a "category of one" dental practice?

It's a dental practice that values the power of distinction versus the cost of blending in. It's one that goes above and beyond for its patients, creating an environment that's difficult—if not impossible—for others to duplicate.

This distinction doesn't just apply to our physical building, however. It's also found in how we treat our patients and in the services we provide. For our patients, we want to give them the kind of smile that doesn't just serve its purpose, but stands out. A "category of one" company is, at all times, a reflection of the utmost quality in all aspects of its operation and it's this type of practice that we aim to exemplify every day.

We encompass our category of one philosophy with our statement of "changing the way you go to the dentist." This is Integrated Dental's brand. It is our vision and our promise, and the entire organization is dedicated to building, communication, and keeping that promise to every single patient.

The Honest Truth: A Statement from Jami, a Veteran Patient Coordinator

In the spring of 2015, I had my initial interview with Dr. Benson at Integrated Dental. Although I had extensive work history in small private practices, I knew from the first time I stepped into his dental practice that this was going to be a professional experience that I had never had before. Dr. Benson's passion for patient care and dentistry can be felt through just his presence in the office. Since day one, he has set the standard that his practice will be a category of one business.

What does this mean to me as a member of the Integrated Dental Team? It means that we are and will always strive to be the best dental practice in Northern Colorado. This is achieved through a constant focus on clinical training and customer service. Dr. Benson invests in each of his employees on an individual level. Team trainings are provided on a quarterly basis and other funds are allocated to each employee to choose certain clinical and self-improvement courses to attend to further their career and add value to the patient experience. In fact, we receive so much additional training in these two focuses, I consider all of us to have earned an additional degree in our specialty.

It is up to private dental offices, like Integrated Dental, to uphold treatment, quality, and customer service standards within our field in the rise of the corporate dental chains. I take pride in my career as I educate our patients on an individual level about their treatment, insurance benefits, and investment in their oral health. I know that when a person chooses Integrated Dental as their dental home, they will receive dentistry performed at a peak clinical standard as well as a consumer experience that rivals that of Nordstroms and Chick-Fil-A, which truly makes us a category of one.

C h a p t e r   2

WHAT IS AN UNHEALTHY SMILE COSTING YOU?

As humans go, our greatest fears are pretty specific: there's extinction, of course, as well as physical injury, loss of autonomy, separation, and ego-death.[1] If you were to put these in order, extinction would be the most powerful, followed by the others in this same order, ending in ego-death, which can also be described as "embarrassment, humiliation, or any other form of strong self-disapproval."

So, where does "fear of dentistry" fall in this? It depends on how you view a dental visit. More than likely, it falls first under the fear of physical injury—that we'll somehow feel pain during our visit. This isn't an uncommon fear. In fact, about 75 percent of all US citizens have

---

1   Karl Albrecht, "The (Only) 5 Fears We All Share," *Psychology Today*, last modified March 22, 2012, https://www.psychologytoday.com/blog/brainsnacks/201203/the-only-5-fears-we-all-share

some degree of fear of the dentist, from mild to severe, with anywhere between 5 and 10 percent of the population experiencing true dental phobia, meaning that they'll avoid a dentist's office at all costs.[2]

What is that "cost," by the way? What is fear costing us when we won't go to the dentist because our gums bleed a little when we brush or because that one tooth is really starting to ache more often?

What are the opportunity costs of fear?

When we look back at things we've done in life that we were initially afraid of, we most often find that those fears were simply built up in our own head.

Take Geoff's story, for instance. At forty-one years old, he was only able to visit a dentist under IV sedation, and had been that way for at least twenty-five years. For Geoff, this severely limited the dentists he could go to, and meant that he only saw them when something was wrong. In this particular case, he arrived at a dental hospital with tooth pain and an examination showed that he had no less than three teeth that needed to come out. After he had them extracted under sedation, however, Geoff was able to undergo therapy that allowed him to slowly ease into a dental office and eventually have a tooth restored and two cavities filled with just a local anesthetic; with no IV and fully conscious.[3]

If Geoff had been able to deal with his fear earlier in life and simply visited his dentist regularly, it's likely he never would have needed such extensive work done. That is, in a nutshell, a whole bunch of opportu-

2   Peter Milgrom, Philip Weinstein, and Tracy Getz, *Treating Fearful Dental Patients: A Patient Management Handbook, 2nd Edition* (Seattle, WA: University of Washington, Cont, 1995)

3   K.I. Wilson and J.G. Davies, "A joint approach to treating dental phobics between community dental services and specialist psychotherapy services – a single case report," *British Dental Journal* 190, no. 8 (April 2001): 431–2, https://doi.org/10.1038/sj.bdj.4800993a

nity costs—by choosing to let fear keep him from the dentist, it cost him twenty-five years of proactive dental visits, tooth pain from lack of treatment, dental damage, and likely the impact to his self-esteem for a quarter of a century because of a poor smile.

When you think back on your own life, it's likely there are more than a few instances where you had to walk through your fear instead of backing away from it—and you probably found out that you'd made it a lot more frightening in your own head than it was in actuality.

Are Bad Teeth Telling Your Life Story?

Your smile tells your life story faster than any other means known to humanity. First impressions are made in milliseconds, and while research is still trying to pinpoint all the details of how we're able to assess people so quickly, we do know that common facial features play an incredible role in other people's initial—and lasting—perception of you.

"A first glance at a person's face often leaves a lasting impression," writes psychologist Vivian Diller in a July 2012 article for *Psychology Today*. "Facial features are more often remembered following initial interactions than people's bodies or even their personality traits."

Diller goes on to note several conclusions that people make based on their first impression of our eyes, nose, skin, and hair, as well as our smile and our teeth, all of which are viewed and assessed in less than a second.

"A person's smile is the feature that elicits the most immediate and positive reaction from others," Diller states. "People who have a spontaneous and natural smile … send an inviting message to others. It says 'come join me, talk to me.'" An unsmiling face, however, can say, 'I'm not interested.' A frown says, 'go away.'"

Teeth, too, leave a strong impression. "While we may not all have dazzling straight pearly whites, having good oral hygiene goes along with the positive impact that a great smile brings," writes Diller. "Severely crooked or yellowing teeth can imply you are a smoker or heavy drinker. Mottled teeth can reflect certain illnesses, poor nutrition, or an eating disorder. Fresh and bright teeth generally suggest that you are someone with a healthy lifestyle and good grooming habits."

Photogenic or Not, Good Teeth Matter

Good teeth are a hot topic on the acting website Backstage.com. In an article titled "Nothing But the Tooth," actors speak to how improvements to their smiles made significant differences in their careers.

"Before I got my teeth whitened, they [casting directors] made comments suggesting that I was not going to be on TV," said actress Sonora Chase. "That has changed."

Actress Jessica Delfino also shared that a quality veneer made all the difference in her performing career, taking her from being self-conscious about a poorly repaired front tooth to having the confidence to take on the "perfection-loving media."

According to Dr. Michelle Callahan, "Whether we like it or not, we are often judged by our appearance...your smile has more of an effect on what others perceive about you than you think."

In a perception study conducted by marketing research firm Kelton, more than a thousand participants were asked to give their honest opinion on the people in a variety of images, and what they found was that those with straight teeth appeared to have more desirable qualities than those with crooked teeth, including the snap judgment that they were "happy" and "professionally successful."

In comparison to people with crooked teeth, the perception study also noted that Americans perceive those with straight teeth as being:

- 45 percent more likely to get a job
- 58 percent more successful
- 57 percent more likely to get a date
- 47 percent more likely to be viewed as healthy

Additionally, close to three in five Americans would rather have a nice smile than clear skin, and 87 percent would give up something for a year if it meant having a nice smile for the rest of their life.

So what story is your smile telling others? And just as importantly, how is that story affecting your *life story* going forward?

"Research clearly shows that having decayed or missing teeth has a strong negative impact on self-esteem," notes psychologist Daniel W. McNeil, PhD. "It also has an impact on employability."[4]

Bad Teeth, No Job

When the American Dental Association took a look at oral health and well-being in the United States in 2015, it uncovered some

---

4   Rebecca A. Clay, "Drilling down on dental fears," *Monitor on Psychology* 47, no. 3 (March 2016): 60, https://www.apa.org/monitor/2016/03/dental-fears

alarming statistics. Young adults were almost neck-and-neck with low income adults in agreeing that "the appearance of my mouth and teeth affects my ability to interview for a job," and one in four adults avoid smiling due to the condition of their mouth and teeth. Judging by what we just learned from psychologist Vivian Diller, this means that a quarter of adults are unintentionally hurting the first impression they give others just because they're too embarrassed to smile.

For a case in point, just look at the story of "Shelly" as reported by the Deseret News in Salt Lake City, Utah.

In 2012, a counseling office in Salt Lake City was looking for a front desk employee and while they were getting plenty of applicants, none met all of their specific qualifications. Then, Shelly arrived at the office as a temp. A thirty-five-year-old mother of three, she was reportedly "pleasant to work with, competent, and kind to the patients." In fact, another front desk employee urged leadership to hire Shelly on permanently. Yet, when her temp position ended, the company chose not to bring her on.

When asked why Shelly wasn't hired, employees were apparently told that it was because she had bucked, crooked teeth.

"He [the office manager] said it wasn't the image we wanted to project at our clinic," said one of the front desk employees.[5]

Image is the New Communication

Communication is becoming more and more image-focused, with social media reflecting this through a massive uptick in video messaging. As of 2017, more than 70 percent of Gen-Z (those born after 1995) spent

---

5   Mercedes White, "No teeth means no job," Deseret News, last modified December 27, 2012, https://www.deseretnews.com/article/865569512/No-teeth-means-no-job-How-poor-oral-health-impacts-job-prospects.html

more than three hours a day watching videos online, and their social platforms of choice, such as SnapChat and Whisper, are almost solely image and video-based.[6]

While most employers aren't as obvious about their motivations in hiring or not hiring certain individuals, you can be certain that a good smile is going to play a big part in other people's first and ongoing impression of you: a factor that a woman in California was well aware of as she sat outside of a state dental clinic overnight.

At fifty-three years old, Patty knew she needed dental work if she was going to land a job. As she waited outside of the clinic, she told an NBC news reporter about her five broken teeth, three cavities and gum abscess, and how the pain was only part of the reason she was there—she knew the condition of her teeth was an important part of the hiring process.

"I really don't smile a lot," she told the reporter. "I know that when you have a job, you want to have a pleasant attitude and you've got to smile and be friendly."

The report went on to quote Dr. Susan Hyde, a dentist and population scientist at the University of California in San Francisco, "If you want to portray someone as being wicked, they have missing front teeth. If they're ignorant, they have buck teeth. Even from a very early age, we associate how one presents their oral health with all kinds of biases that reflect some of the social biases that we have."

Dr. Lindsey Robinson, dentist and president of the California Dental Association, added, "Customer service jobs, good entry-level

6   Nelson Granados, "Gen Z Media Consumption: It's A Lifestyle, Not Just Entertainment," Media & Entertainment, Forbes, last modified June 20, 2017, https://www.forbes.com/sites/nelsongranados/2017/06/20/gen-z-media-consumption-its-a-lifestyle-not-just-entertainment/

jobs … they're not available to people who have lost the basic ability to smile, to function, to chew properly."[7]

But the chain of consequences resulting from bad teeth doesn't stop here. Poor dental health can also affect your immediate health, and apart from making it difficult to work when you're not feeling well, it can affect your long-term wellbeing and can even result in death.

A Heart Attack—and Diabetes, Stroke, and Cardiovascular Disease—Waiting to Happen

In 2007, a twelve-year-old boy in Washington, D.C. died from a toothache. It was a combination of unfortunate circumstances that led to the tragic event, but ultimately, what could have been an $80 routine extraction ended up costing him his life. His family paid close to $250,000 in medical care, including brain surgery in an attempt to save the boy from the infection that had spread from a tooth abscess into his brain.[8]

This is an extreme instance, but the fact is that bacteria, which accumulate quickly in the mouth as they feed on the food particles surrounding un-brushed teeth, have instant access to the bloodstream through the inflamed gums that occur with periodontal disease. These bacteria don't go through any filtering process, either, as they would if they entered the body through the lungs, stomach, ears or nose. In other words, inflammation, the gaps created by a

---

7   Jonel Aleccia, "Bad teeth, broken dreams: Lack of dental care keeps many out of jobs," NBC News, last modified June 12, 2013, https://www.nbcnews.com/feature/in-plain-sight/bad-teeth-broken-dreams-lack-dental-care-keeps-many-out-v18906511

8   Mary Otto, "For Want of a Dentist," Washington Post, last modified February 28, 2007, http://www.washingtonpost.com/wp-dyn/content/article/2007/02/27/AR2007022702116.html

receding gum line, and other untreated dental conditions, are akin to having an un-bandaged open wound on your body. Those bacteria can jump right in and start wreaking havoc, which is why researchers are discovering that there are more diseases than just the obvious ones associated with poor dental health.

- **COPD.** COPD, or chronic obstructive pulmonary disease, is caused by chronic bronchitis, emphysema, or recurring respiratory infection, and has been associated with periodontal disease due to bacterial pneumonia living in the mouth and making its way into the airway.

- **Diabetes.** Periodontitis has been linked to diabetes—both types 1 and 2—so often that it's now being referred to as one of the main complications of diabetes. Reports have suggested that it's a two-way street for these diseases, as well—that diabetics are more likely to get periodontal disease, and periodontal disease may have a negative impact on glycemic control.

- **Heart Disease and Stroke.** Evidence is continuing to grow on the relationship between infectious agents and systemic diseases, with certain bacteria that thrive in dental infections being identified as potentially linked to heart disease. For example, as we said earlier, bacteria or viruses in the mouth can get directly into the blood stream, where they can cause inflammation, blood clots, and narrowing of the arteries.

- **Preterm Birth and Low Birth Weight.** Bacterial infection in the mouth may contribute to adverse pregnancy outcomes, as the harmful bacteria and other toxins created by the infection can get into the blood, cross the placenta, and harm the fetus. Additionally, the reaction of the mother's immune system to the infection could directly or indirectly interfere with growth and/or delivery.[9]

This Isn't Just About Teeth— It's About the Rest of Your Life

This book isn't about promoting dentistry. It's about helping you discover the long-term opportunity costs of fear and the importance of being proactive about the health of your smile.

The first step is understanding the importance of a healthy mouth, which you should have a better idea of after reading this book. The next step? Understanding that when you're not healthy, you're not living at your full potential.

---

9   "Oral Health in America: A Report of the Surgeon General," National Institute of Dental and Craniofacial Research, https://www.nidcr.nih.gov/DataStatistics/SurgeonGeneral/sgr/home.htm.

Chapter 3

UNLEASHING HUMAN
POTENTIAL

At the age of fourteen, Susan still remembers the conversation that took place between her dentist and her parents, when her dentist first urged them to take her to an orthodontist. There was some medical terminology batted about, but one line stuck with her so clearly that she can still hear her dentist saying it today; "If you don't do something now, we'll probably have to break her jaw when she's older."

If she hadn't heard her dentist say that, she might have fussed a little more about the braces her orthodontist fitted her with, but instead she took it all in stride and even switched out her bracket bands to reflect the holidays as they went by. A little over a year later, the braces came off and everyone in the office "ooh"ed and "ahh"ed over her beautiful smile.

Fast forward to a little over two decades later and thirty-seven-year-old Susan couldn't quite remember when she stopped wearing her retainer, though she was sure it was within a year or two after getting her braces off, and certainly before she went to college. Consequently, her teeth had drifted to the point where she could noticeably tell a difference in how they sat in her mouth.

One of the issues people face when it comes to maintaining a healthy smile is the lack of clarity around the natural aging process and its impact on your teeth. Orthodontic relapse is a condition that a lot of post-braces patients fall victim to, and one that we see in the dental office pretty frequently. The issue is that people rarely understand the importance of wearing a retainer and the fact that time and other dental conditions down the road can all affect the hard work that your doctors put into that straight smile so many years ago.

After braces, teeth need at least one year to stabilize and get used to their new positions in the jaw. This is when retainer wear is at its most important—to protect the teeth from relapsing into their former positions and allow them time to solidify in their new positions in the jaws. If a retainer isn't worn, or is worn infrequently, during this time, the teeth may shift and if the patient doesn't visit her dentist, she may not notice that shift for some time.

Even if a retainer is worn for at least a year, after the patient stops wearing it, the teeth once again fall victim to outside—and inside—influences. Teeth grinding, for instance, can place strain on the teeth of the upper jaw, and tooth loss can cause the remaining teeth to drift into the vacant spot. Internal influences could be genetics, which can prompt your teeth to shift, for instance, or gum disease can cause the structure to weaken.

In neglecting her teeth, Susan neglected the potential that her smile could have resulted in. Apart from generally giving her a healthier appearance, straight teeth also create a healthier mouth in actuality—with straight teeth, there are fewer places for food and bacteria to hide, making it easier to brush. And straight teeth that function properly also make chewing easier, which means less strain on the jaw, which means avoiding jaw joint issues down the road.

It's like the old adage "for want of a nail, the kingdom was lost." By not maintaining a healthy smile and being proactive about it, we open the gates to numerous problems down the road. For Susan, drifting teeth meant that they were sitting in less-than-ideal positions in her mouth, making them harder to brush, which meant more bacterial buildup. And more bacterial buildup can cause inflammation of the gums. Inflammation leads to gingivitis, gingivitis leads to periodontal disease and periodontal disease leads to ... well, you read the last chapter, right? It could potentially lead to anything from heart disease to death.

All for the want of proactive, preventative dental care.

Hitting the Reset Button On Your Smile

Unlike many things in life, you have the option of hitting the reset button on your smile. It doesn't matter if you've neglected your teeth, smoked your whole life, or if illegal drug use has caused most of your teeth to rot out—whatever has happened in the past to affect your oral health, technology and advancements in dental science have made it possible to rebuild almost any smile.

We live in a world today where photos are uploaded by the billions every single day. In 2014, for instance, it was estimated that every two minutes, the same number of photos were uploaded to the Internet as existed in the world one hundred and fifty years ago. This is a world where you can no longer hide your smile.[10] The camera is on you constantly and whether or not you realize it, it's having an impact on the course of your life. People make snap judgments based on the images they see of you, and based on their first 0.1 seconds of interacting with you. You're regularly being assessed in situations and under circumstances where you cannot speak for yourself—your image is doing all of the talking.

I'm aware this probably sounds superficial, but regardless of our better efforts, we're still a superficial species. Our instincts still react the same way they did eons ago—an attractive smile still triggers the selection of a mate. It still inclines us to like or trust someone more. Genuine smiles, also called Duchenne smiles—the ones that get you to use those little muscles around your eyes—also signal to others that you're focusing on just them, which in turn encourages them to cooperate with you.[11]

At the same time, the way you feel about your smile also influences your own perception of self. Your self-concept is determined, many times, by the way you look at yourself in the mirror. Do you smile at yourself from ear to ear or do you frown in an effort to conceal your imperfect grin? That perception lives with you and reflects outward, whether you realize it or not, affecting not only your own happiness, but the happiness you could be generating in others.

There is no doubt that a bright and vibrant smile can do more to drive happiness in someone's life than you would think on the surface. When you think about it, what are the things you could do

---

10   Rose Eveleth, "How Many Photographs of You Are Out There In The World?" The Atlantic, last modified November 2, 2015, https://www.theatlantic.com/technology/archive/2015/11/how-many-photographs-of-you-are-out-there-in-the-world/413389/

11   Gil Greengross, "Want to Increase Trust in Others? Just Smile," Psychology Today, last modified April 30, 2015, https://www.psychologytoday.com/blog/humor-sapiens/201504/want-increase-trust-in-others-just-smile-0

in life that will ultimately drive happiness? Most likely, the majority of those things can be traced back to your ability to smile.

What Makes Us Happy?

Research shows that around 40 percent of our own happiness is under our control. So what can you do to make yourself happier - and how do those behaviors relate to your smile?

1. Strong relationships with people you trust
2. Good income / paying bills without stress
3. Taking the time to think about the good things in life
4. Performing voluntary acts of kindness
5. Exercising
6. Living life instead of buying things
7. Living in the moment - mindful meditation
8. Time with friends

Unleashing Human Potential

A lot of people ask me what I do professionally, and when I tell them that I'm a dentist, the typical reaction is, "Oh, you fix teeth."

If only it were that simple.

One of the big reasons I got into dentistry was because I realized the power that a confident, healthy smile can give someone. And I realized that when people have a smile they can be proud of, through cosmetic dentistry, dentures, or orthodontics, they show it a lot more.

I found that the more people smiled, the more confident they were and the easier it was for them to speak and communicate. These people had a higher self-image, and a better self-concept. And believe it or not, I found that the more people smiled, the more career and professional success they experienced and the more productive relationships they had.

So when people jump straight to "you pull teeth" once I tell them I'm a dentist—well, it's not nearly that simple. What I and everyone else in our office are in the business of doing is unleashing human potential. We help our patients regain their ability to smile, and by doing so, we also help them acquire confidence, capability, and allow them to be readier to take on the opportunities in the world and achieve great success for themselves and for their families in the process. In our world, form should follow function. So, if it functions good, it will also look good.

Case Study: What Yearbook Smiles Tells Us

Over the course of thirty years, Drs. LeeAnne Harker and Dacher Keltner followed the lives of one hundred women after graduating from college to determine if a positive emotional expression in their yearbook photo was linked to their life outcomes.

During the study, Harker and Keltner, along with their research team, contacted the women in the study at ages twenty-one, twenty-seven, forty-three, and fifty-two, asking them various questions about marriage, family, and work, among other topics. What they found was that "over time, women who expressed more positive emotion in their yearbook pictures became more organized, mentally focused, and achieve-ment oriented, and less susceptible to repeated and prolonged experiences of negative affect." In addition, they confirmed theories that "individual differences in positive emotional expression were linked to personal stability and development across adulthood, the impressions and reactions from other people, and the marital satisfaction and well-being up to thirty years later, " adding that, "People photograph each other with casual and remarkable frequency, usually unaware that each snapshot may capture as much about the future as it does the passing emotions of the moment."[12]

Overcoming Fear with Practice

Now that you understand the fear, the consequences, and the moti-vation of a healthy mouth, let me share with you how we're working to change the dental experience forever. The first and most important step is education—knowing the *why* behind regular visits to the dentist—but the next is on me and my team, which is to make those visits the absolute best they can possibly be. Doctors can't afford to continue with the old-fashioned model of making patients wait on them. Today, it's the complete opposite. Only those doctors that are willing to put their patients front and center—to cater to *their* needs instead of the other way around—are the ones that are going to survive. And we intend to do more than survive—we intend to

---

12 LeeAnne Harker and Dacher Keltner, "Expressions of Positive Emotion in Women's College Yearbook Pictures and Their Relationship to Personality and Life Outcomes Across Adulthood," *Journal of Personality and Social Psychology* 80, no. 1 (January 2001): 112–124, https://doi.org/10.1037/0022-3514.80.1.112

make your needs our number one priority, and in doing so, become *your* number one dentist.

The Honest Truth: A Statement from Wendy, a Veteran Expanded Duties Dental Assistant

Although my job does provide a paycheck, being a dental assistant has always been a career for me. I love dental assisting and the opportunities it has provided to me to expand my knowledge base, not to mention all the experiences over the course of my journey. That is what this career is to me—a journey. Working with Dr. Benson offers me constant opportunities to serve my patients with compassion, kindness, and understanding. Generally, people do not like visiting the dentist, and I view assisting as an opportunity to make their visit as pain free, anxiety free, and enjoyable as possible. This means serving their needs emotionally while they are here, such as during the procedure, and with comfort items such as a pillow, blanket, headphones or anything else within our means.

I think what people are lacking as consumers in the health care and dental industry today is simple kindness and compassion. I love being able to provide this to our patients at an exceptional level. One specific example of the end result of this philosophy is a patient who needed conscious sedation and nitrous for treatment when she first became a patient. A few months later when she needed additional treatment, she elected to use only nitrous for her procedure. When she returned a few weeks later to conclude her treatment, she was able (by her own choice) to proceed with only local anesthetic—no sedation or nitrous! She was really excited that she was able to overcome her extreme dental anxiety to feeling very comfortable in our office. I attribute this level of trust to the service, kindness, and compassion of the team members involved in her treatment!

Chapter 4

BEST TEAM IN TOWN

Over the years, I have spent a lot of time developing clinical skills, attending advanced training courses and doing everything I could think of to offer my patients the best and most up-to-date care possible. What I was missing, however, was the understanding that my team is the most impactful reflection of my ability. I could go through all the training in the world, but if lackadaisical staff members are treating my patients poorly, that knowledge and experience would never counterbalance that negative first impression.

Today, I understand that we have to stay at the highest possible level of clinical skills, training, and technology, not only to keep up with the rapidly evolving pace of dental technology, but to also provide our patients with the absolute highest quality of service.

The "best team in town" concept is our belief that we should not only have the most competent clinical team on the floor, but also a team that is present in all situations and circumstances, has been trained to stay focused on the patient, and a team that will never compromise on their work. This means that everything from the way appointments are scheduled when you call to how you are greeted when you walk in the door, how you are escorted to the treatment room, and even how you are communicated with should be top-notch and focused only on you.

It's Not a Job, It's a Career

One of our primary goals is to turn each role at our office into a career. This means reinforcing each team member's overall commitment to the practice and the patient, connecting them to the mission of our organization and encouraging them to apply our core values both personally and professionally.

Our Vision Statement

We will be a leader in our field, known for our 5-Star Patient Experience, a highly-educated team, advanced innovation and technology, and community involvement.

Our Core Values

- Inform Before We Perform
- Quality
- Education
- Compassionate
- Trust

Through modeling core values, it is our hope that our staff will have more of a positive impact simply through the behaviors they exhibit, particularly when interacting with patients and with each other.

In other areas, we strive to make a positive impact by providing our staff with the best training, coached in the understanding that we expect from them the highest level of commitment and expectation. As a patient, we want you to understand that we're taking all of these steps to dramatically improve your experience. Our training both in clinical skills and continuing education are not just a "bare minimum" effort, but are undertaken in order to stay ahead of the curve and at the top of our game.

One of these efforts ties directly into our desire to be a Patient-Centric office, which is prompting our staff—and particularly our hygienists—the desire to not just treat the patient, but to be their Oral Health Advocate.

Consider the following feedback I have received from my hygienist after going through multiple patient-centric trainings:

The Honest Truth: A Statement from Shannon, a Veteran Hygienist

The biggest problem that I see with other hygienists in other offices is that they aren't stepping up to the plate to be their patients' Oral Healthcare Advocate ... not just a hygienist. I'm not pointing fingers—some just have not seen or been taught any different.

I have always seen myself as a healthy smile giver. It is my job as a hygienist to help my patients understand that routine oral care can provide a healthy foundation which in turn leads to a healthy smile. I have always informed my patients about what they needed to know regarding procedures and why sometimes going beyond a simple cleaning was necessary. However, when met with resistance, I didn't always know how to handle their irritation, their impatience, and their questions about financing. I never correlated that if I didn't learn how to properly communicate and bypass their opposition, I was not fulfilling my role as their Oral Healthcare Advocate.

As hygienists, if we don't step up for the patient, then we are the ones that are keeping a problem alive that has existed in the dental industry for way too long.

I still remember the first training session Dr. Benson provided our office. We were all skeptical as he assured us this was not going to be the "typical" training. It was not going to be a clinical how-to but more of how to communicate—with our team, our patients, and even beyond the office and effectively communicating with our family.

During our first training session that was centered on our hygiene department, our trainer described the importance of advocating for our patients in such a way that it changed the way I looked at my career forever. From that day on, I was no longer an "oral janitor" but an Oral Healthcare Advocate. My life's purpose is to give my patients healthier smiles and healthier lives, and to get as many other people to join me as possible. As Integrated Dental has grown, and as my position has grown, I have imparted this wisdom on all my fellow hygienists that have joined our team.

What I do is not just a nine-to-five job. It's not just a paycheck. Being a hygienist is our chance to serve—and to save lives. Oftentimes the dental office is the only health care office that a patient sees on a semi-annual basis. As Oral Healthcare Advocates, we can screen for medical conditions such as high blood pressure, diabetes, and certain autoimmune diseases. We are also the only people in our patient's lives that are aware of their oral health. We can't be afraid to tell them what they need to do. Our patients trust us 100 percent to tell them what the best possible treatment is for their oral health condition.

Dr. Benson has taught me about a comprehensive, whole-mouth approach to dentistry through trainings he has provided at our office and through the Dawson Academy. If the muscles in the jaw are not happy, this can lead to other diseases and problems such a migraines and occlusal disease. I have learned about treatment modalities for patients who suffer from these problems through medication and splint therapy. Dr. Benson has also provided me with the opportunity to be a part of a dental community that is different than any I have ever experienced by creating a different experience for our patients at Integrated Dental.

As a hygienist, if you know that a procedure will benefit your patient, but you don't give 100 percent effort in educating them on it, then you are doing that patient a serious disservice. They don't know what you do, but they want to understand and they won't know what to ask unless you give them as much information as you can. By being in the health field industry, we serve our patients by educating them on their oral care and how it affects their overall health.

That's just the honest truth. If you're doing any less, then you aren't fulfilling your duties as a healthcare provider. It isn't that you have bad intentions if you don't—none of us do! Since becoming a hygienist, I've realized that the people in this industry are some of the warmest, most caring individuals I've ever met. However, some hygienists are out there doing the bare minimum of service rather than consistently over-delivering to their patients—being reactive instead of proactive about their treatment. I know that we can do better than that.

During training, our team learned to refocus on what each patient truly needs, and we made it our mission to give him or her the best solution. I now feel empowered to give my patients a healthier life and to take responsibility for that patient like I would a member of my own family.

Continuing Education

In addition to standard and continuing education, our staff may be participating in upward of one hundred hours of training per year on subjects directly related to the customer experience, such as the oral healthcare advocate training the hygienist spoke to earlier.

Our focus is on having a consistent process for everything from the front desk to the hygienists, to dental assistants, to the doctors in the practice. It's these processes that allow us to work with the other professionals in our office so that every patient receives the same, consistent quality of care.

Our Office is a "No Judgment" Zone

Let's address the elephant in the room right now—people judge. They judge us by our appearance, by the clothes we wear, by our opinions, even by the way we cut our hair. That may be able to slip under the radar at other establishments, but that attitude of judgment is left at the door at our office. If any one of our employees walks in with a judgmental chip on their shoulder, then that's the day they lose their job.

We do *not* judge anyone who comes to us. We do not allow any unchecked personal opinions from our team members drive how you are treated. We don't treat you differently based on what type of insurance you have or if you don't have insurance—we're simply interested in understanding what it is you need or want to have done, making sure you're comfortable, and providing you with what you need.

As a doctor, we want our patients to understand that this is not a normal commitment, but it is one that I believe is key to the relationship we share with our patients and the reason why our number one source for new patients today is referrals from existing ones.

Chapter 5

STEWARD OF YOUR SMILE

Let me ask you a question—have you ever worn down your tires and gotten a flat?

If so, what did you do? Did you go to the mechanic and ask for a patch, or did you get a new tire?

A lot of us have opted for the patch—even when the tires are so worn they're practically bald because we tell ourselves that we just can't afford new tires right then. When that happens, however, what do we end up doing? Eventually we have get that new tire, but we're spending more for it because we've had to pay for the patch and any other damage that happened to the car from running on bald tires until we bought new ones.

More often than not, we do more damage and end up costing ourselves more when we choose to "patch" instead of truly repair. Sometimes when a patient has not focused on their oral health, and their treatment plan is extensive, I ask them, "How much do you spend on your car? How often are you in your car?" then I say, "Now, how much are your willing the spend on your health, since you need that 24/7?"

It's the very same situation with your smile. Your teeth bear much of the brunt of your lifestyle. If you enjoy acidic beverages such as coffee, wine or energy drinks, then that enamel is getting worn down every day. If your diet is high in sugar, then your teeth are constantly being bombarded by bacteria, and that's even if you're brushing the recommended two times a day (which a staggering one in five people *do not* do).

Taking care of your mouth is more than just brushing—there's a lot more that goes into it, and yet so few of us are on the preventative side of smile care. For instance, tell me—do your gums bleed when you brush? Do you ever notice a little bit of a gap between your gum and your tooth when you feel around your teeth with your tongue? Or is there buildup on a tooth or two that you just can't get off with brushing?

All of these conditions—gingivitis, receding gum line, and plaque buildup, respectively—are signs you need to see your dentist as soon as possible, and yet so many of us ignore these kinds of issues until they start to hurt. And by then, the conditions have likely progressed to point where more involved treatments may be necessary.

It's the strangest thing! We could go see the dentist every six months, get our teeth cleaned, floss regularly, and let the dentist take care of minor cavities as they occur, or we could do as more than a third of Americans do and just not go to the dentist until those preventative conditions become a severe problem.[13]

Acidic and sugary drinks and snacks aren't the only challenges that our teeth face on a regular basis. There's also the impact of stress on teeth—grinding (also called "bruxism") is associated with anxiety and depression, and can cause you to wear away your enamel and expose the dentin, which is much softer than the enamel and can lead to sensitivity and cavities.[14] It could even cause your teeth to crack and, over the long-term, it can lead to complications with your jaw joint (also called the "TMJ" or temporomandibular joint) and may even cause facial muscles to become enlarged from overuse, potentially blocking your salivary glands, which then can lead to inflammation, pain, and dry mouth … which leads to more cavities, and so on.[15]

We define stewardship as "protecting and growing the owner's assets with fierce intensity." Therefore, taking stewardship of your smile is about recognizing that your health is a valuable belonging, and taking those preventative measures is paramount to maintaining your oral health so you never reach the point of paying $10,000 for a repair that could have been a minor fix if you'd seen your dentist on a regular basis. Our team educates all of our patients on their treatment plan, and explains to them that it is never easier or cheaper to fix it than it is today.

---

13   Lecia Bushak, "Oral Health Isn't Much Of Americans' Concern, Poll Finds: One-Third Didn't See The Dentist Last Year," Medical Daily, last modified April 29, 2014, http://www.medicaldaily.com/oral-health-isnt-much-americans-concern-poll-finds-one-third-didnt-see-dentist-last-year-279468

14   Angelina R. Sutin et al., "Teeth grinding: Is Emotional Stability related to bruxism?" *Journal of Research in Personality 44*, no. 3 (June 2010): 402–405, https://doi.org/10.1016/j.jrp.2010.03.006.

15   Donna Pleis, "Teeth Clenching And Grinding Can Affect Your Dental Health," Bruxism, Colgate, last modified, http://www.colgate.com/en/us/oc/oral-health/conditions/bruxism/article/teeth-clenching-and-grinding-can-affect-your-dental-health-1114

When you do run into those repairs, though, stewardship is also about making the best choice for your smile rather than the cheapest one. Remember the tires analogy? Patching your problem ultimately ends up costing you more than getting it right the first time. And as your dentist, I never want to encourage you to just patch something five or six times when we can eliminate the problem once and for all.

Why Your Insurance Carrier Is Not Important

When it comes to your health and your smile, my first thought is always going to be "What's the right thing to do here?" It's about what we can do to protect you and help you grow and live a full and healthy life. If a close relative comes to me with a dental condition, for instance, I'm not going to tell her how to patch it for now—I'm going to tell her how to fix it for the long-term. And the same goes with my patients—I don't want to recommend temporary repair when you will be far better served in the long-term by fixing it right the first time.

This is why we do not take dental insurance carriers or dental insurance benefits into account when presenting patients with their options for dental treatment. Our office accepts and works with over 90 percent of available dental insurances and we will obtain your benefits to the best of our ability. We will estimate, based on your benefits breakdown, an approximation of what your insurance carrier will pay. However, we do not let dental insurance carriers dictate your dental needs.

It is important to note here that dental insurance works differently than medical insurance. With dental insurance, there is usually an annual benefit maximum ranging from $1,000 to $2,000 per year. Dental insurance also limits the patient annually on the number of exams, dental hygiene cleanings, x-rays, and other necessary procedures, regardless of your physical or oral health. For example, due to some medications patients take, they develop periodontitis and may need more than two cleanings per year to stay healthy. Typically, insurance only allows two cleanings, even though it is medically necessary for the patient to have more. Dental insurance will also "downgrade" certain procedures across all plans and not on a case by case basis. This means that even if you cannot have amalgam fillings (metal) because of allergies, they will still only reimburse for amalgam fillings on posterior teeth because they are the cheaper option. Therefore, the patient must pay the difference in not only what the insurance didn't cover but also the difference in the tooth colored and amalgam filling.

Dental insurance benefits vary among carriers. But more importantly, dental insurance varies from employer to employer. The employer chooses what they want to cover with the dental insurance carrier. Although we strive to estimate a patient's dental portion to the best of our ability, ultimately, every single dental plan is different and what the carrier chooses to cover, or not cover, does not take into account the patient's health history or current health conditions.

Our primary objective is your dental health. We will not limit your treatment based on what a dental insurance company, who does not know you or your health history, says they will "allow." We offer many financing options in our office to assist each patient in obtaining the dental treatment care they need and deserve. Remember, how well you take care of your mouth impacts every aspect of your life from the day you are born and will follow you to the grave.

What Is the Cost of Neglecting Your Dental Health?

Health is an interesting value. It's something we all need and yet, it's not something we can purchase. We can't walk into a gym and say, "Okay, I'll take two well-defined biceps, a washboard stomach and a set of toned glutes. How much will that be?" Instead, we have to work hard to produce and maintain a healthy body on our own. It takes time and it takes discipline, but for the sake of our overall health, it's worth it.

When we say "worth it," what do we mean? There's the personal, innate worth, of course—the cost of time and effort put into brushing our teeth or hitting the gym are "worth" it when it leaves us feeling healthier. But there are also physical financial benefits to good health, as well.

One economics researcher, Michael Grossman put it well when he described human behavior regarding health: "Individuals inherit an initial stock of health that ... can be increased by investment," adding that "Individuals 'choose' their length of life" when investments are made through direct inputs into that stock, such as medical care, diet, exercise, and recreation.

If you really enjoy reading into the process of creating economic models, then you should certainly check out Grossman's paper "On the Concept of Health Capital and the Demand for Health." Otherwise, I'll just get right to one of his conclusions, which is that when we take stock of our life (or, in this case, look at it like investing in stock), we can predict that the more people educate themselves about the benefits of good health, including longevity, the more proactive they'll be about obtaining it.[16]

Consider the following study conducted by a group in Scotland, who set out to determine whether or not a country-wide nursery toothbrushing program was not only making a difference in the longer term dental health of children, but if it was also saving money on dental costs down the road. Specifically, the study looked at the cost savings from improvements in the dental health of five year olds through the avoidance of needing extractions, fillings, or other treatments due to decay.

The first step was determining the complete costs for filling or extracting a decayed primary tooth, and then on average, how many of those dental treatments were conducted over a ten-year period.

They found that not only did the dental treatments for five year olds decrease over time once the toothbrushing program was initiated, but by the program's eighth year, the expected financial savings alone were two and a half times the cost of the program.[17]

How, then, can we be proactive about dental health? With two simple initial investments:

1. Brushing and flossing at least twice a day

2. Visiting your dentist at least twice a year.

That's all the investment you need to make on a stock that can have incredibly rewarding returns.

---

16   Michael Grossman, "On the Concept of Health Capital and the Demand for Health," *Journal of Political Economy* 80, no. 2 (April 1972): 223–255, https://doi.org/10.1086/259880

17   Yulia Anopa et al., "Improving Child Oral Health: Cost Analysis of a National Nursery Toothbrushing Programme," *PLoS ONE* 10, no. 8 (August 2015), http://doi.org/10.1371/journal.pone.0136211

Opportunity Costs of Dental Health

Essentially, an opportunity cost is the choice that you give up when you make a decision. That is, when given the choice between "gum" and "a mint" and you choose "a mint," the opportunity cost is the gum.

When you expand on that idea, "opportunity cost" not only stands for the loss of one choice in preference of another, it also represents the long-term consequences of your choice.

If we stick with the gum/mint choice, for instance, by choosing the mint, we could, say, miss out on the longer-term benefit of chewing gum. If the gum was sugarless and the mint was not, we'd be taking a hit on calorie intake by choosing the mint (as well as doing just that much more potential damage to the teeth thanks to that extended sugar exposure). Extrapolate that even further and maybe chewing gum could have kept us from thinking about eating a snack—but by taking the mint, we experienced a sugar spike and now we're eating a burrito at 2:30 p.m. instead of taking a walk, and by the end of the week, we've gained three pounds.

Opportunity Cost of Dental Health

OPTIONS: *brush and floss teeth everyday* **OR** *don't brush and floss teeth everyday*

CHOICE: *don't brush and floss teeth everyday*

WHY? *because I don't have time*

COST: *new implants to replace the rotten ones*
$3,000 to $6,000 per tooth

Opportunity costs can be subjective, but they can also be quite objective and practical. In this case, consider the opportunity cost of deciding not to brush and floss every day.

The mouth is the perfect breeding ground for bacteria, and not just one type, either—there are close to four hundred different species of microorganisms, mostly bacteria, living on every filmy surface and in every hard-to-brush crevice.

According to dental researcher Sigmund Socransky, "In a clean mouth, one thousand to one hundred thousand bacteria live on each tooth surface. A person who doesn't have a terribly clean mouth can have 100 million to one billion bacteria growing on each tooth."[18]

While a good amount of those bacteria and microorganisms are beneficial, helping to fight off disease-carrying microorganisms that try to enter the body through the mouth, the oral cavity can also house harmful bacteria that, if not brushed away, can eventually irritate the gums, causing gingivitis, which evolves into periodontal disease. At this point, some of the most direct results of poor dental health may occur, including bad breath (otherwise known as halitosis) and tooth loss.

I discussed several of the following related conditions in an earlier chapter, but they're important enough to bring up again as the stewardship of your dental health can quite literally mean the difference between life and death. Those open, bleeding gums provide instant access to the bloodstream, where their presence has been linked to conditions such as:

- **Dementia**: researchers following more than five thousand people for eighteen years found that those "who reported not brushing their teeth daily had a 22 percent to 65

---

18   Jane E. Stevens, "Oral Ecology," MIT Technology Review, last modified January 1, 1997, https://www.technologyreview.com/s/400012/oral-ecology/

percent greater risk of dementia than those who brushed three times a day." Another, smaller study on Alzheimer's has noted that the brains of those with the disease exhibited more bacteria associated with gum disease than those without the mental illness.

- **Endocarditis**: bacterial infection of the lining of the heart and its valves, causing inflammation and infection

- **Heart disease:** wherein harmful bacteria make their way directly to the heart

- **Stroke**: bacteria-related inflammation of arterial walls and blood clotting can cause the arteries to narrow and lead to stroke

- **Rheumatoid arthritis**: periodontal disease can increase the pain caused by this disease

- **Lung disease**: both pneumonia and chronic obstructive pulmonary disorder (COPD) can be worsened by harmful bacteria making its way from the mouth to the lungs

- **Brain Abscess**: as noted earlier in the case of the twelve-year-old who died from a decayed tooth-related brain abscess, bacterial infections of the mouth can be life-threatening if left untreated. [19]

It only takes about three days of not brushing for detrimental conditions to form. Once you pass seventy-two hours, the volume of bacteria will have reached the point where they're producing enough acid to carve holes in tooth enamel, and plaque may have solidified

---

19 Lauren F. Friedman, "13 Awful Things That Happen If You Don't Brush And Floss Your Teeth," Business Insider, last modified February 14, 2014, http://www.businessinsider.com/what-happens-if-you-dont-brush-and-floss-your-teeth-2014-2

to the point where it becomes difficult, if not impossible, to remove without professional intervention.[20]

What, then, is the opportunity cost of choosing not to brush and floss your teeth at least twice a day? It could be the cost of a filling, an implant, dentures, your overall health and even, your life.

Steward of your Smile

In our office, we adhere to the stewardship model, which is to protect you, to help you make good decisions and to help you grow as a person through the things that we can have an impact on.

When it comes to treatment, first and foremost, we believe in being good stewards of our patients, their time, their financial resources, and all of the transactions that occur in our business, which means helping our patients steward over their decisions in a meaningful and productive way. This is because we've found that many non-patient-centric offices will guide their treatment path based upon what they think the ability of the patient is to pay. This is simply *not* the philosophy that we use.

Instead, we treat you as a person and make recommendations to you as though you're a member of our family and allow you to ultimately make the decision that's right for you. We believe in providing you with the best recommendation for your condition, and the only way to do that is to leave the question of funding out of the picture.

As I pointed out earlier, there are times when budgets require people to patch something, be it a leak in a pipe, a hole in a weak roof, or a tire. But when we think about that decision over the long run, patching is pretty much a guaranteed way to have the problem

---

20 Jane E. Stevens, "Oral Ecology," MIT Technology Review, last modified January 1, 1997, https://www.technologyreview.com/s/400012/oral-ecology/

return, and likely in a worse way than the first time around. This is why we like to give patients the option to fix things correctly the first time since it winds up being more cost effective and better for the patient overall.

Take the leaking pipe, for example. Patched, it may work a little while longer, but when it starts to leak again, that leak will likely go unchecked for a certain period of time and eventually cause more damage than it did when it was patched. The cost then ends up being the cost of fixing the problem correctly and repairing the damage done in the meantime. So which is the more cost-effective solution?

Convenient Financial Arrangements

When we consider the financial part of any visit to our office, we always approach it with these words in mind: flexible and without fear. We don't want to avoid discussing it—it's something we'll need to talk about anyway, so why not get it out there? But we don't want it to be awkward or to become a barrier to working with us. For these reasons, we offer multiple options for patient financing, including flexible payment plans.

In all cases, we like to provide our patients with options because there are times when we need to patch, but we always make sure to provide all of the information for the appropriate fix, as well, and discuss financial options if the budget is a problem. Above all, it's important to us that we educate our patients on the conditions resulting from either decision, including the consequences of patching versus fixing something correctly. Ultimately, the choice is in the patient's hands inside of our practice.

The Honest Truth: A Statement from Skye, a Veteran Financial Coordinator

To be a patient-centric financial coordinator is a balancing act. My role is to educate our patients on the financial aspects of their treatment plan, without letting insurance companies or other financial situations dictate what is best for their health. Many times, Dr. Benson will provide the patient multiple options regarding treatment time or treatment plans. This could mean breaking up a large treatment plan into smaller visits that can be spread out over time or creating multiple treatment plan options. Each treatment option will get the patient healthy, however, one is usually the most ideal for functions and esthetics.

I am an advocate for each patient's oral health by educating them on all of their treatment and financial options as I guide them towards the best fit for them personally. I serve our patients by providing them a detailed layout of their financial investment in their treatment plan and educating them on how their particular insurance functions within their plan. Most patients are astounded by how much information our office willingly gives, instead of holding back or hiding financial information like a secret. Dr. Benson and our team truly stick to the philosophy of "we inform before we perform."

Chapter 6

FREEDOM DAY USA: A DAY OF FREE DENTISTRY

One of the foundations of our practice is financial stewardship, and an important part of that is committing to living off of less than you earn, and giving a portion of what we make to the community.

We do this through several activities, including school and athletic sponsorships, sponsoring events with the city of Greeley, an annual Toys for Tots toy drive, Compete to Beat Hunger with the Weld County Food Bank, and more. But one of our favorite events that we plan, coordinate, and participate in, the event where our entire team feels we make the most impact in our community, is our annual day of free dentistry through our Freedom Day USA event.

During our Freedom Day USA event, we provide free exams, x-rays, fillings, extractions, and cleanings to active duty and retired military personnel, veterans, and their spouses. In the past few years, we have had some very generous dental labs donate dentures and crowns as well! This day is not just about our doctors providing free services, but our entire team volunteers the entire twelve-hour day to contribute each of their individual skills to provide for the people who have fought for and defended our freedoms.

Freedom Day USA

Freedom Day USA is the United States of America's largest national THANK YOU movement and was founded by Dr. Robert Martino, owner of Wilson Martino Dental in West Virginia. Dr. Martino's vision was to give members of our military a day of free services, goods, and products to thank them for protecting our freedom. The first annual Freedom Day USA event was held on September 12, 2013, and Integrated Dental was proudly a part of this inaugural, nationwide movement to say thanks.

For Integrated Dental's first event in 2013, I had less than a week to prepare. We closed down the schedule to regular patients, and a few radio stations assisted us and made a few announcements about Freedom Day USA the morning of the event. My small office consisted of myself, one assistant, two hygienists, and one patient coordinator and we saw sixteen patients and gave away over $15,000 in free dentistry! I had not even owned Integrated Dental for one year, but I knew then that each year Integrated Dental would hold this event, and each year it would be my favorite day of the year.

After the first event, we realized we could make a bigger impact if more dental offices partnered with us for our local Freedom Day USA event. Dr. Ralph Reynolds, from Reynolds Oral and Facial Surgery, and Dr. David Richter, from Richter Orthodontics, and their teams joined our event in 2014 and have volunteered every year since. We have also been joined by other incredible doctors through-out northern Colorado including doctors and teams from Northern Colorado Endodontics, Premier Endodontics, and Rocky Mountain Smiles. Local and national dental laboratories have even contributed certificates for free dentures and crowns. Local restaurants including Cables Pub and Grill, Bulldog Pub & Grub, and Wing Shack, and bakeries such as Just Piped Bakery and Kels Cookie Jar have always ensured that our volunteers remain fed and energized and that our patients have something to snack on while they wait. Every year our list of volunteers has grown with people who want to offer their time and talent to our service members.

My team is truly passionate about helping others. In 2017, 815 businesses, including 362 dental offices in 46 states, volunteered nationwide for Freedom Day USA, giving away millions of dollars in free dentistry. Each year, more businesses have joined our thank you movement in Greeley making it bigger and better. Our mission is to continue this tradition as both our community and our office grows. It is exciting to think about that as a combined effort with all the dental teams and local businesses that have participated with us in the annual event, we have provided over $350,000 in free dentistry in six years to our servicemen and women of our community.

The Impact of a Free Day of Dentistry

Here are some testimonials from some of our Freedom Day USA patients. Their words can express the impact of this event much better than mine can.

> "Dr. Benson and the team at Integrated Dental Arts have a special place in my family's heart! My husband is a Navy veteran and district 6 teacher, so we have little

money to spend on medical and dental care. Often my husband and I would forego our dental needs and even the annual cleanings and exams because we could not afford them. Dr. Benson and his team have made it their mission to thank vets in our area for their service to our country by providing dental care to them and their families. I cannot tell you what a blessing this has been to our family! We now look forward to Freedom Day each year, making it a family day to hang with Dr. Benson and his team! I am forever grateful for the service Integrated Dental Arts has given my family and I. Their kindness, smiles, and dental work are appreciated by this Navy veteran's family!"
—Jessica, proud Navy vet wife

"I woke up one day and my teeth were killing me, so I called my case manager with the VA and they told me that Integrated Dental Arts had paired with two other doctors and were hosting a day of free dental care to active and retired military personnel. Their office is located in Greeley, Colorado, over two hours from my house. My step-dad and I got to the office at 2:00 p.m. and the staff was so professional and nice. They sat me in the chair and looked at my teeth and told me they were giving me a new set of dentures AT NO COST. Three and a half hours later, all my teeth were gone and I had my mouth prepared for dentures. This is a true act of kindness from Dr. Benson and Dr. Reynolds. I want to say thank you to their staff for their professionalism and kindness. I want to share this act of kindness with the world. Thank you!"
—Rudy V.

The Honest Truth: A Statement from Kaela, a Veteran Expanded Duties Dental Assistant

I never had volunteered my time before I started working at Integrated Dental. My first Freedom Day was 2015 and I have had the privilege of participating every year since. Not only are we able to give our service men and women comprehensive dentistry but we have given many of these veterans confidence back. Freedom Day to me means no American left behind, and that is something Dr. Benson and his wife Jenny Benson have helped me come to realize. The skills we have been given are meant to be shared, and the lives we are able to touch along the way is what makes it beautiful.

Low-Income Adults and Poor Dental Health

Qualifying for dental benefits and coverage at the VA is very difficult for veterans and their families. There are numerous eligibilities, but some only provide very basic services, and many veterans do not tick the correct boxes when it comes to receiving care. For instance, to be eligible for full dental benefits covering any procedure, the veteran must have a "service-connected compensable dental disability or condition," be rated 100 percent disabled, or the veteran must be a former prisoner of war.[21]

---

21 "Health Benefits," U.S. Department of Veterans Affairs, https://www.va.gov/healthbenefits/resources/publications/hbco/hbco_faq.asp.

Many patients, veterans included, choose to go to the emergency room when they have tooth pain—especially when they don't have dental coverage or benefits. According to the American Dental Association (ADA), "most hospitals don't have the facilities or staff to provide comprehensive dental care. So many patients receive only antibiotics or pain medication, but the underlying dental problem is not addressed. In too many cases, the patient returns to the emergency room with the same problem—or worse."[22]

Preventable Dental Emergencies

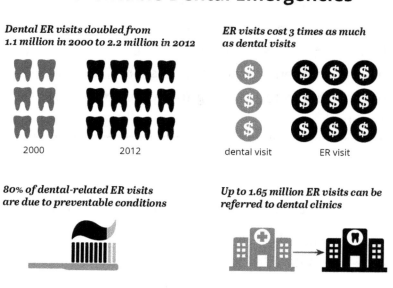

Dental ER visits doubled from 1.1 million in 2000 to 2.2 million in 2012

2000   2012

ER visits cost 3 times as much as dental visits

dental visit   ER visit

80% of dental-related ER visits are due to preventable conditions

Up to 1.65 million ER visits can be referred to dental clinics

Source: American Dental Association, ADA.org

Emergency room visits for dental pain have increased significantly over the years, with 2.1 million visits in 2010. Most of these were for non-traumatic dental conditions, and a 2015 ADA report

---

22   "From the Emergency Room to the Dental Chair," American Dental Association, http://www.ada.org/en/public-programs/action-for-dental-health/er-referral

estimates that up to 79 percent of dental-related ER visits could have been diverted to dental offices.[23]

The ADA goes on to point out that an increasing number of adults are forgoing regular dental care for a number of reasons, including the fact that dental benefits coverage has continued to decline for working-age adults.[24]

"The problem, while worse among lower income brackets, affects people across the economic spectrum," the ADA states, which is just one reason why programs such as Freedom Day USA are becoming increasingly important.[25]

How We Participate

In 2017, Freedom Day USA events across the United States had 815 business, including 362 dentists, in 46 states provide millions of dollars in free dentistry, goods, and services to our servicemen and women. At our practice, we strive to help as many people as we can during our free day of dentistry event. Our event is broken into two days in the fall; our Freedom Day USA Registration Day is in September, where patients can register, fill out their health history, and have their dental x-rays taken. Our Dental Services Day is in October, where all volunteer offices schedule appointments and

23   Thomas Wall, Kamyar Nasseh, and Marko Vujicic, "Majority of Dental-Related Emergency Department Visits Lack Urgency and Can Be Diverted to Dental Offices," American Dental Association's Health Policy Institute, August 2014, http://www.ada.org/~/media/ADA/Science%20and%20Research/HPI/Files/HPIBrief_0814_1.ashx

24   Thomas Wall and Marko Vujicic, "Emergency Department Use for Dental Conditions Continues to Increase," American Dental Association's Health Policy Institute, April 2015, http://www.ada.org/~/media/ADA/Science%20and%20Research/HPI/Files/HPIBrief_0415_2.pdf?la=en

25   "From the Emergency Room to the Dental Chair," American Dental Association, http://www.ada.org/en/public-programs/action-for-dental-health/er-referral

complete as much of the registered patient's necessary dental work as we can.

Additionally, we're committed to donating 10 percent of our revenue each year to this event and other worthy causes.

In 2019 and beyond, our goal is to encourage more dental facilities, labs, and specialists, as well as more local businesses, to participate in our event. We welcome all volunteers, even if they do not have dental experience. For more information on Freedom Day USA, please visit www.FreedomDayUSA.org, and to learn more about our local Freedom Day USA event, please visit our website at www.IDA-Greeley.com.

Chapter 7

BEGIN WITH THE END IN MIND

Did you know that, between the ages of twenty and sixty-four, adults average about seven lost permanent teeth? And about 10 percent of Americans between the ages of fifty and sixty-four have *no* teeth left?[26] That's a lot of tooth loss, and if you're thinking right now that this average loss is probably greater on the older adult end than the younger adult, consider the following statistics from the American Dental Association's Health Policy Institute:

- Young adults are the most likely to report problems due to the condition of their teeth and mouth.

- 35 percent of young adults have difficulty biting and chewing

---

26 Lauren F. Friedman, "13 Awful Things That Happen If You Don't Brush And Floss Your Teeth," Business Insider, last modified February 14, 2014, http://www.businessinsider.com/what-happens-if-you-dont-brush-and-floss-your-teeth-2014-2

- 33 percent of young adults avoid smiling due to the condition of their mouth and teeth

What was also surprising about that report was that only 37 percent of the adults participating in the national survey reported that they'd visited the dentist in the last year, and only 77 percent planned to visit one in the coming year. This, despite the fact that just about all of them (95 percent) agreed that regular dental visits keep them healthy and a majority (82 percent) believed that a straight, bright smile will help you get ahead in life.[27]

Okay, enough statistics. What it comes down to is that dental health is incredibly important at every age, and at every stage in your life, you risk dental health issues. As we age, the risk rises, which is why it's our job to remind you that the decisions you make about your dental health today are going to stay with you for the rest of your life. If you neglect your teeth now, chances are that you'll need more work later down the road and if you neglect those bigger repairs, then you might end up being one of those ten-percenters without any teeth whatsoever.

Coming back to the importance of good stewardship, not only is it beneficial to see your dentist regularly, but it's also important to know the kinds of dental conditions that you can expect with age as your teeth wear, and as any work you've had done begins to break down and your gums begin to recede.

For instance, I've been shocked to have people come in that undoubtedly need a crown on a tooth, and yet they accuse me or my staff of making up the fact that they need it. But if you think

---

27   "Oral Health and Well-being in the United States: Data & Methods," American Dental Association's Health Policy Institute, 2015, http://www.ada.org/~/media/ ADA/Science%20and%20Research/HPI/OralHealthWell-Being-StateFacts/Oral- Health-Well-Being-Methods.pdf?la=en

about how cavities are cared for—cleaning out the diseased area and bonding in a filling every five to twenty years, depending on conditions—then after two, three, or even four decay removals and filling replacements, inevitably there won't be much tooth left to fill and a crown will be necessary.

We don't want this or any procedure to be a surprise to you. Instead, it is our job to teach you about the natural progression of dental care and at what stages you may expect to take some extra preventative steps to keep your mouth healthy over the long term.

You can eliminate a lot of pain, discomfort, and frequent visits to the dentist by being proactive about your dental health. Our goal is to educate you so that you never feel that we're trying to "get" you to do something you don't want to do.

Check out the chart on page 85. There, you can jump to the most common dental conditions that are occurring at your age. I would suggest that you read it so you can have a good understanding behind any of the suggestions we make to you the next time you visit our offices. If you choose not to take preventative measures, that's your decision to make. However, know that if you choose to neglect your teeth for long periods of time, then you should budget to fix your teeth and take care of any related health conditions that may arise because of that neglect.

The best way to think about this is to begin with the end in mind. As you near the end of your life, what kind of teeth do you want to have? If you're like most people, then what you want is to have real teeth and a real smile. And you can have that - if you first understand that it is your responsibility to achieve it.

When I first became a dentist, my wife's grandfather, affectionately known to everyone as Big Daddy, came to my office as a new patient for his dental health visit and comprehensive exam. I asked him what his dental goals had been and what they continue to be. He said, "Buddy, I want to die and be buried with all of my natural teeth. I've made it this far. I feel like I am doing pretty good." He was eighty-eight at the time. He never missed a dental check-up, even while serving in World War II, after retirement, or after I became a dentist. When Big Daddy passed away at the young age of ninety-eight, he was only missing one of his natural teeth. His health, including his oral health, was his goal and he made it his responsibility to achieve it.

As dentists, we're simply your partner and a provider of solutions to help you achieve your goals. It's on you to take the actions necessary to make those goals happen.

Part Two

Your Mouth at Every Age

Dental Expectations at Every Age

Childhood
Ages 0-6
Teaching proper toothbrushing
Treating common dental emergencies
• Knocked out tooth
• Cracked tooth
• Tongue or lip bite
• Toothaches
• Objects stuck in teeth
Fluoride treatment
Ages 7-9
First orthodontic visit
Establishing proper eating habits—avoiding sugary drinks and foods
Applying dental sealant (painted on child's 1st & 2nd molars as they emerge)

Pre-Teens and Teenagers

Reinforcing proper eating habits

Greater likelihood of cavities

Hormonal impact on oral health

Ages 20-39

Increased risk for gingivitis

Risk of TMD pain due to:

- Tooth movement or other dental conditions
- Injury
- Craniofacial muscle spasms
- Rheumatic disease
- Other factors that cause the temporomandibular joint to shift

Stress impacts on oral health

- Tooth grinding
- Cracked teeth

Maintaining orthodontic adjustments (such as wearing a retainer after braces)

Ages 40-59

Increased risk of periodontal disease

Maintaining annual comprehensive periodontal evaluation

Old cavities may have to be crowned, or the tooth removed/replaced

Increased risk of obstructive sleep apnea

Maintaining preventative dental care

Ages 60+

Risk of cavities and tooth loss increases

Risk of gum recession

Risk of dry mouth

Reapplying fluoride varnish

Dental implants and dentures

Impact of osteoporosis on oral health

Watching out for signs of oral cancer

Dental care and dementia

Dental concerns may seem to come up completely out of the blue, but more often than not, they've been around for a while—we either just didn't notice them before or chose to ignore them until the irritation or pain become too much to bear. That's one of the biggest problems with dental issues—you could have a cavity and not even realize it until it becomes so deep that it hits the nerve. Or you may have gingivitis and ignore that tinge of blood when you're brushing or flossing until it becomes a full on case of periodontal disease.

This is what I sometimes call the "treadmill of dental life." Decisions regarding your dental health can come at you so quickly that you have to make rash decisions that you don't want to make—such as extraction or surgery—because of the condition you're in. However, if you're consciously taking preventative actions on the front end, then that treadmill slows down and you either don't have to make those decisions, or you have a lot more time to consider your options because you're aware of the condition long before it becomes a serious issue.

In this section of the book, we'll look at many of the dental concerns that can occur over a lifetime and what you can be doing now to prevent them. Or, if you haven't taken preventative measures for some time (such as brushing regularly and seeing your dentist at least once a year), this section should give you an idea of what conditions to expect at your current life stage.

Chapter 8

CHILDHOOD

Everyone has a childhood memory of what their first dental visit was like, which is why parents today are looking to make that experience better. They want their kids to look forward to seeing the dentist, which is why one of the first things we tell new parents is to bring their children in by the age of three, unless otherwise directed by a pediatrician.

That may seem a little young, but think of this way: when babies are born, their mouths are sterile. Within hours, however, they're colonized with organisms that will stay with them for the rest of their life. These bacteria, protozoa, viruses, and yeasts are mostly harmless, but once they settle in, they start building a habitat that's more welcoming to other, less-harmless organisms. Once a baby cuts those first teeth, the bacteria that's most likely linked to tooth decay—*streptococcus mutans*—is also likely to make an appearance.[28]

One of our biggest concerns when a baby's teeth first start to come in is that of Baby Bottle Tooth Decay, also known as "bottle rot." This condition typically affects the upper front teeth and is caused by prolonged exposure to sugar-containing drinks—including milk (milk contains 12 grams of naturally occurring sugar per cup, otherwise known as lactose). Prolonged exposure can occur when a child is put to bed with a bottle, or if they use a bottle as a pacifier, and that sugar is the best way to activate the rapid growth of *streptococcus mutans*.

When sugar is present, *S. Mutans* feeds on it, releasing acids that can eventually eat away at tooth enamel, making room for plaque to grab ahold, which bacteria latch onto and from there, begin forming new holes. The more sugar that's added, the more this condition spreads until the mouth's natural cleanser—saliva—can no longer wash it away.

Even though a child will eventually lose his or her baby teeth, these first teeth play a very important role in life. They are needed for developing clear speech, chewing, and will also help the adult teeth come in correctly. I have often told my own children that their baby teeth are their "practice teeth" to learn how to brush properly and develop healthy dental habits.

---

28   Jane E. Stevens, "Oral Ecology," MIT Technology Review, last modified January 1, 1997, https://www.technologyreview.com/s/400012/oral-ecology/

Toothbrushing and Dental Health Care for Ages 0–6

Infants

- For babies whose teeth have not emerged yet, use a clean, damp pad or washcloth to wipe your child's gums after each feeding.

- Only place formula, milk, or breast milk in bottles. Do not fill them with juice, sugar water, or soft drinks. Do not put an infant to sleep with a bottle. Bottles should be finished before nap time and bedtime.

- If an infant uses a pacifier, only give them a clean one—do not dip it in honey or other sugar-containing liquids.

1–3 years old

- When your child's teeth come in, use a child-size toothbrush and no more than a pinch (about the size of a grain of rice) of children's toothpaste to brush their teeth until three years of age.

- Encourage drinking from a cup.

- Encourage healthy eating habits.

- Ween your child from their pacifier once real food has been introduced.

3–7 years old

- Brush your child's teeth with a child's toothbrush and a pea-sized amount of children's toothpaste.

- If your child wishes to brush his or her own teeth, make sure to supervise the process to ensure that all of the teeth are brushed and all of the toothpaste is spit out instead of swallowed. Supervision should occur until the child is between the ages of six and seven.[29]

Dealing with Common Dental Emergencies

As many times as you've warned your child not to climb on top of the monkey bars, or open containers with his teeth, or ride his bike too fast (I could go on, but if you're a parent, you know what I mean), dental emergencies still occur. Here are a few ways to deal with them when they come up:

- **Knocked-out tooth**: try to put the tooth back in its socket without touching the root. If you can't, then either place the tooth in your child's cheek next to the gum, or if you're worried about the child swallowing the tooth, place it in a glass of milk. Then call your dentist immediately.

- **Cracked tooth**: rinse the mouth with warm water to clean it out and give the child a cold compress to place against the side of the mouth to keep any swelling down. Then call your dentist immediately.

- **Tongue or lip bite**: rinse the mouth with warm water and apply a cool or cold compress to the affected area.

- **Toothaches:** rinse the mouth with warm water and gently use dental floss to remove any food caught between teeth,

---

29 "Baby Bottle Tooth Decay," Mouth Healthy, American Dental Association, http://www.mouthhealthy.org/en/az-topics/b/baby-bottle-tooth-decay

as this can be exacerbating the pain. Call your dentist as soon as it is convenient.

- **Objects stuck in the teeth:** try to use floss to gently remove it, but if that does not work, call the dentist. Do not try to use a sharp, solid instrument to remove the object as it may cause further damage.

"Colorado Brown Stain" and the Introduction of Fluoride

You've probably heard me or other dentists talking about the importance of using toothpaste containing fluoride at every age, including those first toothbrushing years. There are a lot of reasons behind this, first and foremost that, while fluoride is added to tap water, very few people drink tap water anymore, opting instead for bottled water or filtered water (note, however, that "activated carbon" filters do not remove fluoride. Only processes such as reverse osmosis and deionization can remove the mineral).

Secondly, bottled water can be incredibly acidic. A study published in the *Journal of Dental Hygiene* found that, of the fourteen commercial bottled water brands tested, ten were acidic, with a pH of less than 7.

"Dental professionals continually educate patients on the dangers of consuming acidic food and drink due to their potential to contribute to dental erosion and tooth decay," the study noted, "However, water is not typically categorized as acidic." In investigating the pH values as reported on each of the bottled water manufacturers' websites, the researchers also found that the actual values were lower (more acidic) than those reported.

So why is fluoride added to water?

The discovery of fluoride and its dental benefits ironically began with the problems that fluoride was causing. In 1901, a young dentist named Frederick McKay arrived in Colorado Springs, Colorado, with the intention of opening a dental practice. What he found when he arrived was astonishing—the residents of the town had dark brown stains on their teeth, some so significant that "sometimes entire teeth were splotched the color of chocolate candy." Eventually, the condition became known as Colorado Brown Stain.

Apart from the coloration, however, the staining didn't seem to be causing any harm, and in fact, after years of research, McKay found that these mottled teeth were very resistant to cavity formation. Additionally, he found that city residents whose permanent teeth came in and calcified before the stains set in did not develop the stains later, so the staining had to occur while the teeth were developing.

It was later discovered that incredibly high levels of fluoride in the water were causing the brown stain—a condition that became known as "fluorosis." But lower levels of fluoride didn't stain and actually appeared to be beneficial. Later on, studies confirmed that fluoride ions easily absorb into the surface of teeth where demineralization has occurred, and bond with the enamel.

The bonded fluoride then attracts other minerals, such as calcium, to the damaged area, thereby strengthening the tooth overall.

The next question to answer, then, was how the benefits of fluoride could be used without triggering the ugly staining caused by fluorosis. Decades after the cause of fluorosis was discovered, Dr. H. Trendley Dean, head of the Dental Hygiene Unit at the National Health Institute, began to study exactly how much fluoride needed to be in water before fluorosis occurred, and whether or not physically and cosmetically safe levels of fluoride in water would help fight tooth decay.

In 1945, Dean worked out a deal with Grand Rapids, Michigan, to safely fluoridate the town's drinking water over a fifteen-year period. After eleven years, Dean was able to confirm that children born in Grand Rapids after the fluoride was introduced were 60 percent less likely to develop cavities.

Today, fluoridation projects benefit more than 200 million Americans and fluoride can be found in just about every toothpaste brand on the market.

Ages 7–9: First Orthodontic Visit

The best time for a child's first orthodontic visit is between the ages of seven and nine. This may seem like an odd time since most children still have quite a few of their baby teeth at this age, but this is actually the perfect age to have a preliminary screening done to ensure that there are no issues developing, such as crossbites, over-, or under-bites.

If there is an issue, this age is also the ideal time to start Phase One Treatment, which focuses less on the teeth and more on changing jaw growth. The younger a child is, the easier it is to guide the jaw into a stable, ideal bite. Less than 20 percent of children need Phase One treatment. Imagine how much more growth a seven-year-old has ahead of him or her, rather than a twelve or thirteen-year-old—when potential issues are caught during this window of opportunity, orthodontists can get a jump on corrections and reduce the amount of time that child will need to spend in braces later on. There is also the airway to consider. Does your child snore? A properly trained dentist can recognize these issues and refer appropriately.

Ages 6–12: Dental Sealant

Dental sealants are thin coatings painted on a child's first and second molars (which emerge around the ages of six and age twelve, respectively) that fill in the deep grooves of the tooth to prevent cavities. According to the Center for Disease Control (CDC), "once applied, sealants protect against 80 percent of cavities for two years and continue to protect against 50 percent of cavities for up to four years." This is particularly important as the permanent back teeth are where nine out of every ten cavities occur.

*Top Three Tooth-Rotting Beverages**

Sports Drinks

Sweetened Iced Tea Drinks

Energy Drinks

*People always say "Don't drink soda because of the sugar" but the truth of the matter is that a sugar-free energy drink is worse for your teeth than a classic cola, because it's more acidic. It's that combination of sugar and acid that does the most damage, but acid is ultimately worse on your teeth than sugar.

Chapter 9

PRE-TEENS AND TEENAGERS

The pre-teen years are when you really reinforce the importance of brushing teeth twice a day on their own. At this point, your child should have already had their first orthodontist visit and may or may not be undergoing treatment to prevent a bite condition. Of all the things you can do for your child's dental health at this age, having sealant applied is one of the most important, if only for the long-term impact that this pretty simple process can have.

Eating for a Healthy Mouth

When it comes to maintaining overall mouth health, diet and nutrition are just as important as good brushing habits. Diet (the food we eat) and nutrition (the nutrients in the food) both impact the health of our mouth differently. Diet has a local effect, impacting the integrity of our teeth, saliva, and the mouth's pH balance, while nutrition has more of a systemic effect, impacting the integrity of the jaw bone, teeth, and supporting structure of the teeth. That is, changing your diet will more directly affect your mouth health while changes in nutrition will also have an impact, but it will happen over a longer period of time and affect the greater structure of the mouth.

Where we often run into trouble is the overconsumption of what's called "fermentable carbohydrates," which are those added and naturally occurring sugars in food. The difference between fermentable carbohydrates and other carbohydrates is that the fermentable kind breaks down in the mouth instead of later on in the digestive tract, sticking around to feed bacteria and launch the decay process.

Fermentable carbohydrates come in obvious and not-so-obvious forms. There are those foods that definitely contain sugar, such as candies, cakes, cookies, sodas, and chocolates. And then there are the less-obvious: bread, breakfast cereal, bananas, crackers, potato chips, pretzels and even dried fruit.

Additionally, the "stickier" these fermentable carbs are, the worse they are for your mouth, as they latch on to the nooks and crannies of the tooth and feed the bacteria that produces the acid that eats away at tooth enamel. "Sticky" doesn't just mean gooey and gummy in the way raisins and licorice are sticky—it can also mean "gets stuck easily" in the way potato chip crumbs can become wedged between your teeth and stick around long after you've finished eating them.

What are the best foods to eat for a wholesome diet, good nutrition, and an overall healthy mouth? The Dietary Guidelines created by the US Department of Agriculture and the Department of Health and Human Services is a great place to start:

A healthy eating pattern **includes**:

- A variety of dark green, red, and orange vegetables
- Legumes (peas and beans)
- Grains, at least half of which are whole (brown rice, oatmeal, whole wheat bread)
- Fresh, whole fruits
- Low-fat or fat-free dairy, including milk, cheese, yogurt
- Protein foods, including seafood, poultry, eggs, lean meat, nuts, seeds, and soy products

A healthy eating pattern **limits** saturated fats, trans fats, added sugars and sodium, and includes consuming:

- Less than 10 percent of daily calories from added sugars
- Less than 10 percent of daily calories from saturated fats
- Less than 2,300 mg of sodium per day

If alcohol is consumed by adults of legal drinking age, it should be limited to one drink per day for women, and two drinks per day for men.

Every diet should begin with a strong base of grains as well as a daily intake of:

- 2 1/2 cups of vegetables
- 2 cups of fresh fruit
- 3 cups of calcium-containing milk, yogurt, and/or cheese
- Proteins (meats, beans, eggs, nuts)

And when it comes to snacking, try to choose non-sticky, non-fermentable carbohydrates. For example:

Best choice:

- Cheese
- Protein (meats, beans, eggs, nuts)
- Milk products (no sugar added)
- Water

Okay choice:

- Whole fruits such as apples and pears (these contain natural sugars, but have enough water in them that the sugar is diluted and saliva can more easily wash them out of the mouth)
- Vegetables (while vegetables contain carbs, they don't have enough to be dangerous)
- Unsweetened carbonated waters (these often contain a small amount of sodium)

Worst choice:

- Candy
- Cookies

- Crackers
- Bread
- Muffins
- Potato chips
- Pretzels
- Dried fruit
- Bananas
- French fries
- Cakes
- Soft drinks and other drinks containing sugar, including fruit juices

Ages 13–19: Treating Cavities

When lunch consists of a trip to the convenience store or a vending machine for a soda and a candy bar, cavities are eventually going to be an issue. A lot of teenage boys are full on into not taking care of themselves, and while girls tend to do a better job of taking care of themselves and their dental health, cavities can still become an issue—particularly if you have a family history of dental conditions.

Even though kids should already be seeing their dentist twice a year, this age range is when a bi-yearly checkup becomes incredibly important. Cavities need to be caught early and treated before they lead to further tooth decay.

Again, one of our philosophies is that it is never easier or cheaper to fix a dental problem than it is today. This is especially true of small cavities. I am aware that many kids do not look forward to going to the dentist, and they like shots even less, but encouraging a child to fix a dental issue now can save them pain and discomfort later. It will also foster healthier dental habits in the future.

When it comes to fillings, preference in the United States has more or less shifted away from silver amalgam and toward composite fillings, though there are a number of filling options available, and the procedure itself is pretty simple.

Types of Fillings

Depending on your preferences, the extent of tooth decay, and whether or not you have any allergies to certain materials such as metals, there are a number of options for filling materials, including:

- **Gold**: While expensive, gum tissues actually tolerate gold incredibly well and the fillings can last in excess of twenty years. However, apart from the cost, gold fillings also take longer as they often have to be made to order by a third-party lab before they can be cemented into place. This can require multiple visits before the procedure is complete.

- **Silver (amalgam):** Also a material that's pretty resistant to wear, silver fillings also tolerate the heat and moisture of the mouth well, are relatively inexpensive, and last an average of fifteen years. However, since they're dark in color, they're more noticeable. Compositionally, most silver fillings are composed of mercury, silver, tin, copper, and other trace metals. Sometimes a silver filling is necessary for clinchers and grinders or for areas that cannot be kept dry enough for tooth-colored fillings to bond.

- **Composite:** This is increasingly the most used filling type as the color is much closer to the natural color of the tooth. However, they tend not to last as long as metal fillings, with an average lifespan of three to ten years depending on care, and common liquids such as coffee and tea can cause them to stain. "Composite" is short for "composite resins," which is usually a combination of specialized plastics and a filler such as silica.

- **Porcelain:** Like gold, porcelain inlays typically need to be custom created by a lab and then bonded to the tooth. These fillings can be matched to the exact color of the tooth and can last between fifteen and thirty years. By nature, porcelain is also resistant to staining. These fillings, however, can be cost-prohibitive, with prices similar to the cost of gold fillings. Many times, our office can complete these on our E4D machine in the office in one day, so we do not have to send them out to a laboratory.

Basic Filling Procedure

1. The process of cleaning and filling a cavity begins with local anesthesia, which is used to numb the area around the tooth so you don't feel pain during the process.

2. Then we clean out the decay using a small drill and shape the space so the filling will fit in tightly. If we're doing a bonded filling, we'll also etch the tooth with an acid gel before placing the filling.

3. Finally, we'll place the filling and polish the tooth to ensure that the filling is smooth and comfortable as well as fit to the opposing teeth in a way that will not further damage surrounding tooth structure.

Cavities by Age

How likely are you to need dental care as you age? Check out these statistics from the United States National Health and Nutrition Examination Survey (1999 - 2004) on the percentage of adults in each age range with either a cavity, or missing or filled permanent teeth:

Ages 20–34: 85.58 percent
Ages 35–49: 94.30 percent
Ages 50–64: 95.62 percent

How Puberty (Hormones) Can Affect Your Teeth

Along with all the other changes your body goes through during puberty, one of the more overlooked ones is the change that happens with your gums.

Between the ages of eleven and thirteen, when puberty is most likely to occur, gum tissue becomes more responsive to the accumulation of dental plaque and may bleed and become inflamed more frequently. When these symptoms become more prevalent, the condition is generally referred to as chronic marginal gingivitis, or puberty gingivitis, and it's generally believed to be caused by the increased hormone levels that occur with puberty*.

Both males and females are susceptible to the condition, and its onset is believed to be predictive of the formation of more significant periodontal diseases later in life.

This is just another reason why good dental health is incredibly important in the pre-teen and teenage years, as proper oral hygiene today can be the difference between healthy teeth and gums for a lifetime.

*Of note, the hormonal changes that can occur with pregnancy and menopause have also been associated with an increased risk of gingivitis and periodontal disease.

C h a p t e r   1 0

AGES 20–39

The college years are another span of life where cavities are more likely to appear. The typical college diet doesn't help, with late-night study snacks coming into play more often and the general neglect of leafy green vegetables in one's diet. College is also when gum disease starts to pop up, starting out with the light bleeding of the gums during brushing, which is caused by gingivitis. If left untreated, those irritated, inflamed gums can quickly evolve into full on periodontal disease.

The good news is that gingivitis is pretty reversible during this age range. If you can get back into regular dental visits, regular cleanings, and brushing your teeth at least twice a day, the inflammation can go away without any permanent damage. If, however, the gingivitis goes for too long untreated, then not only will your teeth need to be cleaned, but your gums, as well, which is a much bigger deal. Think of it as similar to the condition that your car would be in if you didn't wash it for five or six years. You can't just drive that kind of buildup through the car wash and expect it all to come off—you have to get some serious detail work done.

What are the signs of gingivitis?

That little bit of blood in your toothpaste every time you spit? That's not supposed to be there. Gingivitis is the swelling and irritation of the gingiva, which is the part of your gum at the base of your teeth, and if it's not taken care of quickly it can lead to tooth loss, periodontitis, and other serious gum diseases.

Apart from a bit of blood when you brush, other signs and symptoms of gingivitis include:

- Puffy, swollen gums

- Dark red gums

- Tender gums

- Bad breath

- Receding gumline[30]

Gingivitis begins most often with poor dental health. When the biofilm on teeth isn't brushed away regularly, it can build up to form plaque, and that plaque is what causes irritation. Then, as the plaque builds, it turns into calculus—otherwise known as tartar—which is much more difficult to remove than plaque and is a breeding ground for bacteria. Only a professional dental cleaning can remove calculus. If that calculus isn't addressed, it will begin to irritate the gingiva, causing irritation, which then allows the gums to bleed more easily.

---

30 "Gingivitis," Mayo Clinic, https://www.mayoclinic.org/diseases-conditions/gingivitis/symptoms-causes/syc-20354453

This bleeding then opens the door to more bacteria getting directly into the gums and the bloodstream, leading to tooth loss, periodontitis and the risk of those diseases we mentioned earlier.

What increases the risk of gingivitis?

Poor brushing habits are the most common risk factor for gingivitis, but other conditions can contribute to the risk, including:

- Dry mouth

- Poor nutrition

- Dental restorations that don't fit well

- Crooked teeth that aren't cleaned well

- Conditions that cause a decrease in immunity such as HIV/AIDS, leukemia, or cancer treatment

- Smoking or chewing tobacco

- Old age

- Hormonal changes

- Genetics

- Viral and fungal infections

Headaches or TMJ pain or both?

Of all of the hinging points in your body, the temporomandibular joint (TMJ, commonly called the "jaw joint") works harder than any other. Also, due to the combination of sliding motions and hinging, the TMJ is also the most complicated joint in the body. The jaw joint is where all of the major movements of your skull are centered and it is constantly moving, whether you're aware of it or not. On a conscious level, its active when we chew, speak, or yawn, and on a subconscious level its constantly making micro movements such as clenching, grinding, shifting, and repeatedly opening and closing.

Due to its connection to the trigeminal nerve—the largest of the twelve cranial nerves which run throughout the upper and lower jaws and into the teeth, eyes, and even the tongue—the smallest misalignment can have a significant impact on the rest of the system.

There are numerous conditions that may lead to facial pain or TMD (tempororomandibular disorder), many of which become more prevalent as we age. These include:

- **Tooth movement or dental conditions** – tooth movement as we age, the wearing down of teeth, and tooth replacement, as well as dental procedures that change how our teeth interact, can affect the TMJ

- **Injury** – trauma to the jaw joint, head, or neck can have long-term effects that may not be felt until months or possibly years after the initial injury occurred

- **Craniofacial muscle spasms** – caused by injury or medications

- **Rheumatic disease** – this condition, which refers to a larger group of conditions that cause inflammation, pain, and stiffness of the joints, such as arthritis, can affect the TMJ as a secondary condition.

Common signs of TMD issues:

- Facial aches and pains
- Frequent headaches
- Tooth wear

- Numerous dental problems (broken teeth, crowns or history of several root canals)
- Aches and pains around the ear
- Tender or painful jaw
- Discomfort or difficulty chewing
- Popping, clicking or grinding noise in jaw joints
- Difficulty opening and closing mouth due to locking of jaw joint

---

A significant sports injury in your teenage years or early twenties, or a car accident that seemed to only result in a case of whiplash, may evolve into issues with the TMJ later in life as the damaged jaw joint deteriorates under the tension of the unbalanced system.

What causes TMJ Pain?

Any time your bite changes, it affects your TMJ, and anytime your TMJ shifts, it can put mechanical stress on your teeth. Think of it like a finely tuned engine—if anything becomes misaligned, however slight, it will put stress on the system. As the stress increases over time, the misalignment becomes worse until the whole system becomes noticeably and painfully out of alignment.

Patterns of dental problems on the back teeth in particular can be a sign of undiagnosed TMJ issues. These problems can include root canals, missing back teeth, cracked teeth, broken porcelain fillings, etc, any of which can indicate that the system is under more stress than it should be. Additionally, teeth that are under additional stress from excessive bite force are also more likely to suffer periodontal problems.

One of the biggest problems with TMJ issues is how long they take to manifest. If headaches due to an injury that affected the TMJ don't appear until years after the incident, then it's not likely that the person suffering from them is going to make that connection.

Good dentists should be on the lookout for these types of conditions. If the alignment of the patient's jaw seems off, even if it's just slight, and we suspect a TMJ or muscle issue, then the first thing we'll do is test the diagnosis. This typically involves the patient being fitted with a type of mouth guard called an occlusal splint, which sets the jaw joint back into an ideal bite when worn. This will relieve the stresses on the joint, resulting in less pain.

An occlusal splint may look like a standard mouth guard, but it does more than just protect the teeth from grinding together at night. Instead, it is custom designed to hold the jaw in just the right position so that the teeth are aligned, relieving the muscle stress being placed on the TMJ by the misalignment, and allow freedom of movement of the lower jaw.

After a few days of wearing the splint, the patient will come back in and we'll discuss the impacts, if any. If the patient is feeling forty or fifty percent better just from wearing it, then we know we're headed in the right direction. If they still feel the same and the headaches aren't getting any better, then we'll continue to fix the tooth issues that they originally came in to see us about and we'll likely refer that patient to another doctor. While TMJ issues are an often looked-over source of headaches and facial pain, other causes include ear infections, facial neuralgias (nerve-related facial pain), and sinus problems.

If the occlusal splint *is* making a difference, then the patient may wear it for anywhere from a couple of months to a couple of years until the jaw settles back into proper alignment.

Home Care for TMD

If you suspect that you have TMD, there are some steps you can take at home to relieve the discomfort:

- Ice packs applied to the side of the face, particularly just in front of the ear where the TMJ is located
- Make conscious efforts to keep your face relaxed with lips together and teeth apart
- Eat softer foods
- Take small bites and chew with both sides of the mouth
- Don't rest your chin in your hand
- Don't bite hard objects, such as pencils, fingernails, cuticles, etc.
- Don't hold phones between the neck and shoulder
- Avoid excessive or extensive movements of the jaw, such as big yawns or chewing gum.
- Practice stress-relieving techniques
- Do gentle jaw stretches or jaw massages. One approach is to place your thumb or fingertip in the small "notch" located about one inch in front of your ears and on the underside of the cheekbone. Gently pressing inward and upward in this spot and rubbing in soft circular motions may provide some relief.

If the TMD pain continues, there are other options for treatment, though each should only be considered after assessing all of the pros, cons, and risks with your doctor:

- **Pain medication:** muscle relaxers, tricyclic antidepressants, pain killers and other medications as prescribed may help with the temporary relief of TMD pain.

- **Dental adjustments:** this involves making changes to the teeth to bring the bite back into balance, called equilibration.

- **Botox:** Since Botox works by blocking the nerve signals to the muscles, it may provide temporary relief to sore jaw muscles when used in small doses, although this method is not approved by the FDA for use with TMJ issues.

- **Surgery:** While surgery is an option, it should be avoided where possible as there are no long-term clinical trials showing the effectiveness of surgical procedures helping with TMJ disorders, and the treatment is often irreversible.

- **Implants:** Artificial implants to replace jaw joints are also an option, but should also be taken under the same strict considerations as surgery.

For more information on discussions around TMJ treatments, visit the National Institute of Dental and Craniofacial Research's page on TMJ disorders: https://www.nidcr.nih.gov/oralhealth/Topics/TMJ/TMJDisorders.htm

Stressed Out? Your Teeth are Probably Feeling the Pressure

"I sheared off my front tooth," actress Demi Moore explained to *Tonight Show* host Jimmy Fallon during a show back in June 2017. "I'd love to say it was skateboarding or something really kind of cool, but I think it's something that's important to share because I think it's literally, probably after heart disease, one of the biggest killers in America, which is stress."[31]

While stress doesn't immediately cause your teeth to fracture, loosen, or fall out, it can cause this kind of damage over time, with stress increasingly becoming more prevalent in younger generations.[32] Under high stress, people may forget to brush or floss, and may not have the time or even think to visit the dentist. The same conditions can also lead to increased cortisol levels in the body, and while cortisol in the short term has an anti-inflammatory effect, extended or exaggerated stress response can lead to cortisol dysfunction, which can result in widespread inflammation and pain.

Stress in America - Harder on Young Adults

According to the American Psychological Association (APA), stress is becoming more of an issue for younger generations (Millennials born between 1984 and 2004, and Gen-Xers born between 1964 and 1984), who report feeling the most stress and the least relief compared to older generations. As of the APA's 2015 stress survey, adults in America:

- Report stress levels higher than what they believe is healthy (3.8 on a 10 point scale)

- Rate their average stress level as 5.1 on a 10 point scale (up from 4.9 in 2014)

---

31   Bruce Lee, "Demi Moore Lost Two Teeth To Stress, Here's How It Can Happen," Forbes, last modified June 15, 2017, https://www.forbes.com/sites/brucelee/2017/06/15/demi-moore-lost-two-teeth-to-stress-heres-how-it-can-happen/

32   "2015 Stress in America," American Psychological Association, http://www.apa.org/news/press/releases/stress/2015/snapshot.aspx

- Were more likely to report experiencing at least one symptom of stress (78 percent vs. 74 percent in 2014)
- Were more likely to report experiencing extreme stress (24 percent vs. 18 percent in 2014)
- Reported higher incidences of illness, with:
  - 67 percent receiving a diagnosis of at least one chronic illness
  - 16 percent diagnosed with depression (up from 12 percent)
  - 13 percent with anxiety disorder (up from 9 percent)
  - 32 percent with high blood pressure (up from 24 percent)
  - 58 percent with obesity
- Millennials and Gen-Xers were more likely to rate money as a stress source
- 45 percent of Millennials say their stress levels have increased in the past year
- 39 percent of Gen-Xers say their stress levels have increased in the past year
- Young adults are more likely than other generations to engage in stress coping/management activities, yet one in four young adults say they don't feel they're doing enough to manage their stress.

Stress can also lead to bruxism, which is the medical term for teeth grinding. If you apply enough force to your teeth, over a long enough period of time, you can do significant damage. On average, a human can bite down with two hundred pounds of force per square inch, which is actually pretty powerful, and when you apply that kind force regularly on just about anything, it's going to cause some damage.

To understand how that kind of pressure affects the mouth, consider how this part of the body is composed. The tissues surrounding the teeth, for instance, are basically tight strands similar to guitar strings, holding everything together. But when you put excessive pressure on guitar strings, what happens? They pop, which is basically what is happening to the tissues around your teeth when you clench and grind. This is why the gums start to recede around teeth affected by bruxism, as the forces cause those tissues to break. If those forces continue, they go on to wear away the enamel, exposing the dentin and creating access points for bacteria to get directly into the blood stream.

Bruxism can occur consciously or subconsciously, while you're awake or asleep, and may not seem to be a concern for months or even years after it first starts to occur.

Signs of bruxism include:

- Dull headaches (especially in the morning)

- Sore jaw muscles

- Pain radiating from the ear

- Teeth sensitivity

- Chipped, cracked teeth

- Loose teeth

- Damage on the inside of the cheek from chewing or biting

- Indentations in the tongue

While bruxism is common in younger children, the condition is usually temporary and more likely due to allergies, teething, or misaligned baby teeth as opposed to stress. Most children outgrow teeth grinding by their teens.

If bruxism continues, or if you suffer from it as an adult, then the long-term pressure and grinding of the teeth can lead to chipping, cracks, and loose teeth that may eventually fall out, as well as the wearing down of the enamel. In severe cases, the enamel can become so worn that the underlying layer of dentin is exposed. This not only causes sensitivity, but the dentin, which is nine times softer than enamel, is much more susceptible to decay.

In rare cases, long-term bruxing can lead to the enlargement of facial muscles, which can block the salivary glands, leading to swelling, pain, inflammation, and dry mouth. And dry mouth alone is a major trigger for cavity formation as the lack of saliva means that the mouth doesn't have its natural means of regular cleansing available to it.

While stress can certainly result in bruxism, teeth grinding can also be related to sleep issues and a sign of undiagnosed sleep apnea. To ensure proper care for the patient's long-term health, a sleep study should be done prior to fabricating an oral appliance or completing any permanent dental work. In milder cases, bruxism may not necessarily need treatment. But if the problem persists to the point of discomfort, jaw pain, and damage to the teeth, then one or multiple forms of treatment may be recommended.

Treating Teeth Grinding (Bruxism)

Dental treatment

Although dental treatment may help to relieve the effect of bruxism, it won't necessarily treat the cause. Some options include:

- **Mouth guards and occlusal splints**: mouth guards can protect your teeth from grinding directly against each other while you sleep, and occlusal splints can be custom built to keep your teeth in an ideal bite position, as well as prevent direct contact of teeth during sleep.

- **Dental correction**: if the degree of bruxism has led to teeth becoming so sensitive that you can no longer drink hot or cold liquids or chew properly, then the teeth may need to be reshaped and restored in order to repair the damage.

Behavior modification

If stress is a likely cause of bruxism, behavioral medication and management may help:

- **Stress management**: learning strategies that promote relaxation such as meditation, may help to reduce anxiety, which may have a positive impact on bruxism.

- **Behavior modification**: if you're aware of bruxism and how it's manifesting in your jaw habits, then you may be able to change that behavior by practicing proper jaw positioning, as demonstrated by your dentist.

- **Biofeedback**: through the use of electrical sensors, you can view information on how your body is reacting to subtle changes, which may help in reducing those actions that result in bruxing. For instance, learning how to consciously control your breathing and heart rate can be a helpful calming technique, and learning how to effectively relax the mouth and jaw muscles may reduce the effects of bruxism, or help to eliminate it altogether if it's main source is stress and muscle tension.

- **Lifestyle modifications:** some at-home methods for reducing the factors that contribute to bruxism can include:

  □ Taking relaxing baths, listening to soothing music or exercising

  □ Avoiding stimulating substances such as alcohol or coffee in the evening

  □ Getting a good night's sleep

  □ Asking your sleep partner to let you know if they hear you making any grinding noises, or if your jaw is clicking at night, so you can inform your dentist or doctor

  □ Schedule regular dental exams to spot signs of bruxism early

By addressing teeth grinding earlier in life, you're more likely to avoid its longer-term impacts, and more likely to make it into your later years with most, if not all, of your natural teeth.

Retaining that Smile

While this book isn't meant to focus on orthodontics, a lot of what happens as part of your orthodontist visits directly affect your dentist visits, and vice versa. For instance, if you had braces as a teenager, it's likely that your dentist played an important part in keeping your teeth clean between orthodontist visits, and reporting any concerns, breaks or other conditions to your orthodontist.

After the braces come off, that relationship between orthodontist, dentist and patient continues as the patient is monitored to ensure that the braces did what they were intended to do—and a big part of that has to do with whether or not the patient is good about wearing a retainer.

It's a tough ask for a teenager who just got out of braces to continue wearing another appliance, but the first year after braces is vital for ensuring that the teeth are secure in their new locations. This is why your orthodontist likely recommended that you wear your retainer up to twenty-two hours every day for the first three to six months, then every night at least for the following six months. Most kids are pretty good about that extra year—its the time afterward that presents the most challenge.

If you wore braces as a kid, you should still be wearing your retainer at least three nights a week and ideally every night for the rest of your life.

This is because, even with all of that time in braces, your teeth are going to shift. It may take a couple decades, but your teeth will gradually shift forward and inward with age—unless you have gingivitis or periodontal disease, in which case your teeth will shift much sooner than that.

If, by chance, you have been wearing your retainer regularly since your teenage years, then the other caveat of maintaining that healthy straight smile is getting your retainer replaced as needed; every two to ten years, depending on how rough you are on them. This isn't just because the retainer can wear out, however—it's also because of the inevitable tooth drift that occurs as you get older. Even with retention, teeth are going to shift slightly and the retainer will need to be adjusted in order to keep those teeth in proper alignment. And if you need a new set and you no longer live near your old orthodontist, don't worry—any orthodontist can have a new one made for you.

Over the course of a lifetime, you may go through several retainers, but wearing a retainer at night a few nights out of the week is a small price to pay for the long-term benefit of keeping your teeth straight and healthy.

Chapter 11

AGES 40–59

For most of us, that feeling of invincibility that we've had our whole lives is likely starting to wear off in this stage—and our systems are starting to wind down a little along with it.

On the brighter side, this is the stage of life where a lot of us start taking better care of our bodies. Before this age, parents in particular were putting their children's health ahead of their own, making sure the kids went to the doctor and dentist regularly while neglecting their own health. Once the kids start to grow up, however—and in some cases, move out of the house—moms and dads start to reinvest in making themselves look and feel better, working on getting their looks as close to—or better than—they were in their pre-kid days. This likely means more working out and more time at the dentist, looking into what can not only be done health-wise but also cosmetically.

Unfortunately, this is also the age when people who were neglecting the signs and symptoms of gingivitis are now likely suffering from full-on periodontal disease.

What is Periodontal Disease (Periodontitis)?

Periodontal disease occurs when gingivitis isn't treated, and the gums pull away from the teeth, forming spaces that then become infected. In fact, the word "periodontitis" means "inflammation around the tooth." As the infection grows, the toxins and the immune system begin to break down the bone and tissues holding the infected teeth in place, eventually leading to tooth loss.

The signs and symptoms of periodontal disease are the same as gingivitis—as are the risk factors. Treatment, too, follows the same path, beginning with a complete deep cleaning that involves scraping the tartar from above and below the gum line, and removing rough spots on the tooth root where germs gather. In some cases, a laser may be used to remove all of the offending buildup.

Antibiotic and antimicrobial medications may also be recommended after a deep cleaning (also called scaling and root planning), but if the damage is too extensive, surgery is most likely the next step.

Surgical Treatments for Periodontal Disease

There are two main types of surgical procedures for periodontal disease. Depending on the extent of the damage, your dentist may recommend:

Flap Surgery

This procedure involves lifting back the gums to remove extensive tartar deposits, followed by suturing the gums back into place so that everything fits tightly. Once healed, the gums should fit snug around the tooth and the teeth may appear longer as a result.

Bone & Tissue Grafts

Sometimes flap surgery isn't enough, however, particularly when the disease has eaten away at the gum tissue and even the bone underneath. Bone grafting involves placing a piece of natural or synthetic bone in the area of bone loss in order to stimulate growth. In some cases, guided tissue regeneration may also be used, which involves placing a piece of mesh between the gum and bone that blocks the gum tissue from growing where the bone should be, giving the bone and connective tissue time to grow. A graft of soft tissue may also be used for gum loss, with synthetic material or tissue from another part of the mouth being used to cover exposed tooth roots.

The success of either procedure is entirely dependent on the patient, his or her risk factors and how well mouth health is maintained at home going forward.[33]

Believe it or not, one out of every two Americans over the age of thirty have some stage of periodontitis, which the more advanced form of periodontal disease. And in adults over the age of sixty-five, the prevalence is a little over 70 percent of all Americans.[34]

---

33 "Periodontal (Gum) Disease: Causes, Symptoms, and Treatments," National Institute of Dental and Craniofacial Research, last modified September 2013, https://www.nidcr.nih.gov/OralHealth/Topics/GumDiseases/PeriodontalGumDisease.htm

34 "CDC: Half of American Adults Have Periodontal Disease," American Academy of Periodontology, https://www.perio.org/consumer/cdc-study.htm

Half of American Adults have Periodontal Disease

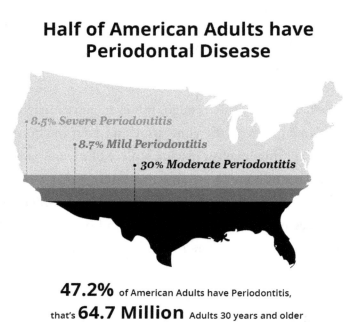

8.5% Severe Periodontitis

8.7% Mild Periodontitis

30% Moderate Periodontitis

47.2% of American Adults have Periodontitis,

that's **64.7 Million** Adults 30 years and older

Source: American Academy of Periodontology/Centers for Disease Control

Interestingly enough, according to study conducted in part by the Centers for Disease Control (CDC), men are more likely than women to have periodontal disease (56.4 percent vs. 38.4 percent in women), and those at the highest risk include current smokers (64.2 percent), those with less than a high school education (66.9 percent) and those living below the federal poverty level (65.4 percent).

"Periodontal disease is associated with age," stated Paul Eke, MPH, PhD, lead author of the study and CDC epidemiologist, "and as Americans live longer and retain more of their natural teeth, periodontal disease may take on more prominence in the oral health of the U.S. Adult population. Maintaining good periodontal health is important to the overall health and well-being of our aging population."

With these findings, co-author Robert Genco, DDS, PhD, believes that periodontal disease should be elevated to the level of Public Health Concern. "We now know that periodontal disease is one of the most prevalent, non-communicable chronic diseases in our population, similar to cardiovascular disease and diabetes," Genco stated.[35]

Have You Had Your Annual Comprehensive Periodontal Evaluation?

According to the American Academy of Periodontology, every dental patient should have a comprehensive periodontal evaluation conducted on annual basis to gauge periodontal health, diagnose existing disease, assess risk for disease, and determine any needed treatment. This service can be conducted during a regular dental visit by the general dentist, or by a dental hygienist or periodontist.

Crowning Moment

If you've had cavities since you were a kid, then crowns are very likely in your near future. Between the ages of forty and sixty is when most fillings have run their effective course. If you've been keeping up with your dental visits, then a cavity that you had filled in your pre-teens or teens was likely redone in your twenties or early thirties. Depending on the original size of the cavity, the redo of that filling will likely take away significantly more of the surrounding structure. Then,

---

35 P.I. Eke et al., "Prevalence of Periodontitis in Adults in the United States: 2009 and 2010," *Journal of Dental Research* 91, no. 10 (August 2012), https://doi.org/10.1177/0022034512457373

when the cavity needs to be replaced again in, say, ten to fifteen years, then there's a good chance that there won't be enough tooth structure left for a filling, and a crown will need to be placed instead.

The fact of the matter is that if you have a cavity, you're going to end up with a crown. It might be sooner, if the cavity is bigger or if you are particularly rough on your teeth, or it might be later—but it's almost always necessary.

Snoring Problem or Obstructive Sleep Apnea?

While obstructive sleep apnea can occur at any age, the risk factor increases with age and the condition is more prevalent in men over the age of forty. While this may not seem like a condition that you would immediately think to bring up with your dentist, we're actually in one of the best positions to help with this disorder as treatment often involves adjusting the jaw in order to open up the airway and increase airflow.

Obstructive sleep apnea, or OSA, is a medical condition in which the sufferer stops breathing for seconds up to minutes at a time while sleeping. These pauses in breathing, called "apneas," can occur thirty or more times in an hour, and breathing often starts again with a loud choking sound or snort. This disruption may not entirely wake the person up, but it will move them from a deep sleep to a light slight sleep, which greatly reduces the overall quality of their sleep and leads to excessive daytime sleepiness.

Even though OSA is a common condition, it often goes undiagnosed as those who suffer from it don't realize it's occurring unless someone tells them. And if a sleep partner does notice, they often write it off as loud snoring instead of something more. If you're concerned that someone is suffering from OSA, the best way to tell is by listening for that pause in breathing between snores. Snoring is usually only a split-second closure of the upper airway that doesn't interrupt the sleeper, while OSA sufferers will noticeably stop breathing before starting again.

Along with that audible pause, other signs and symptoms of the condition include:

- excessive sleepiness
- fatigue
- memory impairment
- mood disturbance
- decreased libido
- social withdrawal
- cardiovascular disease
- lower jaw is too small or is set too far back
- presence of hypertension
- BMI of 30 or higher
- neck circumference of 17 inches or larger
- observed choking or gasping during sleep
- inattention and changes in energy levels during the day
- enlarged tonsils and/or adenoids
- worn down teeth

There is also evidence that people who suffer from bruxism—teeth grinding—may also have some degree of OSA as that jaw movement may be related to the subconscious effort to keep the airway open during sleep, moving the jaw around or clenching the it in order to activate the throat and neck muscles and keep the airway open.

Diagnosing Obstructive Sleep Apnea

The method for determining if someone is suffering from sleep apnea is typically two parts: a basic sleep screening followed by a sleep study conducted with a polysomnograph, or PSG.

The sleep screening can be conducted at the dentist office and usually involves a series of questions or situations to determine someone's daytime sleepiness scale. Two of the more well-known surveys are the Epworth Sleepiness Questionnaire and the Berlin Questionnaire.

Questions on these tests might include gauging the chances that you'll doze off (not feel tired) in situations such as:

- Watching television

- Sitting and reading

- Sitting inactive in a public place such as a meeting

- As a passenger in a car for longer than one continuous hour

- Sitting and talking to someone

- Sitting quietly after a lunch without alcohol

- In a car while stopped for traffic

Other evaluative methods include assessing sleep habits as well as taking physical factors into account, as is the case with the

STOP-BANG Questionnaire, with the name of the test standing for "snoring, tired, observed pressure, body mass index, age, neck circumference, and gender."

Additional evaluation methods could include a cephalometric analysis, to identify any growth abnormalities that may be affecting breathing, a Cone Beam CT Analysis to measure minimum airway volume, an intraoral evaluation to check for any potential visible obstructions, or a take home sleep monitor to measure key parameters like blood oxygen saturation, apnea and hypopnea episodes, and disturbed breathing patterns.

If one or more of these screenings do confirm the risk of OSA, the next step is a supervised sleep study monitored by a polysomnograph (PSG).

While a PSG will measure dozens of factors while the patient is sleeping, one of the most important factors it will be measuring is the person's apnea-hypopnea index, or AHI. This measurement determines exactly how many apneas, or pauses in breathing, the patient experiences in an hour, as well as moments of shallow breathing called hypopneas. Additionally, the study will count the number of respiratory effort-related arousals that patient experiences within an hour's time.

These measurements, along with accounts of the patient's heart rate, airflow, air pressure in the esophagus, oxygen saturation, snoring, eye movement, and even carbon dioxide levels of the skin, are taken into account before presenting the patient with a diagnosis.

Treating Obstructive Sleep Apnea

This is where dentists can play a significant role in treating or even curing OSA. If the condition is caused by a restricted airway, then the patient may benefit from oral appliance therapy.

There are several options for oral appliances that help with sleep apnea, and all of them are designed to hold the lower jaw forward, which creates a larger space between the base of the tongue and the back of the throat. If a patient is experiencing constriction at night, this adjustment should help keep that area clearer.

However, since oral appliances generally rely on the teeth to do their job, they're not recommended for people with periodontal disease or TMJ issues, as the appliance may exacerbate the condition. There are also potential side effects of long term usage, including:

- dry mouth

- excessive salivation

- tooth discomfort

- gingival irritation

- jaw muscle tenderness

- TMJ discomfort

- changes in bite due to teeth shifting from the pressure placed on them by the appliance.*

*This last side effect can often be managed by wearing a tooth positioner—a device that resembles a large sports mouth guard—for twenty to thirty minutes per day to keep the patients' teeth in their original position.

If oral appliances aren't an option, then the most common treatment for the condition is a continuous positive airway pressure device, or CPAP, which blows compressed air into the patient's nose and/or mouth while sleeping. While the CPAP is considered the "gold standard" for OSA treatment, it's also the least tolerated, as the mask can be uncomfortable to wear, and the pressure on the airway can irritate the nasal and upper airway tissues. Other options for treating sleep apnea, apart from lifestyle and behavior modification (losing weight, avoiding sleeping on the back, avoiding alcohol and/or sedatives before bed, etc.), may include:

- **Upper airway electrical stimulation**: a device that can be implanted in the chest to deliver mild electrical impulses to the nerve that controls the tongue, stimulating it to move when the patient stops breathing.

- **Maxillomandibular (double-jaw) advancement surgery**: for patients with significantly narrow airways, surgically moving the upper and lower jaws forward can help to open up the airway and tighten the muscles and tendons in those airways, reducing the risk of airway collapse.

- **Tonsillectomy and Adenoidectomy**: patients presenting with sleep apnea during childhood are more likely to benefit from these procedures, and have been shown to be highly effective in treating pediatric OSA.

- **Tracheostomy**: this procedure creates a small opening in the trachea below an obstruction in the airway. This procedure is usually only done in extreme cases of OSA, when no other options are available.

- **Nasal procedures**: if sleep apnea is mainly due to restrictions in the nasal area, surgeries can be conducted to address the blockage.

- **Uvulopalatopharyngoplasty**: This is a big word for an interesting procedure, which involves removing a portion of the soft palate around the uvula (that fleshy tissue hanging down in the back of the mouth) in order to open up the airway. While this can help with snoring, however, it's typically not as effective as other surgeries and therapies for treating OSA.

Now Is the Best Time for Preventative Dental Care

It never hurts to remind yourself that your dental health down the road depends on how healthy you keep your teeth today. As you age, any problems you have today are going to get worse unless they're treated, and neglect today can result in new issues and problems tomorrow. Overall health can go downhill fast, and keeping your mouth young in old age requires diligence; brushing and flossing twice a day are more important than ever, and keeping regular dental appointments will ultimately cost you much less in the long run, as failing to see the dentist could mean bigger—and costlier—dental conditions down the road.

In addition, remember those conditions that have been linked in one way or another to overall mouth health—diabetes, heart disease, stroke and respiratory problems have all been tied to the risk of bacteria from gum infections slipping directly into the bloodstream and triggering inflammation in organs and tissues.

Want to make it into your golden years with as many of your own, real teeth as possible? Then today is the best day to start a proper dental care routine that will last you the rest of your life.

Chapter 12

AGES 60+

Cavities and lost teeth are a serious issue at this age, in part due to the long-term wear and tear on gums and teeth that has already taken place.

With an average bite of two hundred pounds of pressure per square inch, the human mouth is pretty powerful, but that power also has the ability to wear down on the outer layer of tooth enamel over time. And when you combine a lifetime of chewing and grinding along with exposure to damaging acidic foods and drinks, you run the risk of more cracks, breaks, cavities and overall damage due to that weakened enamel.[36]

---

36 "The aging mouth – and how to keep it younger," Harvard Health Publishing, Harvard Medical School, last modified January 2010, https://www.health.harvard.edu/diseases-and-conditions/the-aging-mouth-and-how-to-keep-it-younger

Gum recession, too, is more common in older adults, with a little more than 70 percent of people over the age of fifty showing some degree of recession, and 90 percent with signs of recession over the age of eighty.[37] When this condition is left untreated, the exposed root is more susceptible to gum disease, which could eventually lead to the destruction of the gum tissue and even the bone around the teeth.

Although there's not much you can do to stop the natural wearing down of tooth enamel, keeping up with daily dental health habits such as brushing, flossing, and regular dental visits are as important as ever at this age.

Toothbrushing a Challenge? Go Electric!

Daily habits that we used to do without a thought can become more burdensome in our later years. Just brushing teeth, for instance, can be difficult if arthritis or other disabilities affecting motor skills are beginning to manifest. For those with limited dexterity, switching from a manual toothbrush to an electric one can make a big difference. Additionally, switching to fluoride toothpastes that aid in the remineralization of the teeth can help strengthen tooth enamel and fill in the weak areas that plaque tends to cling to.

Dry Mouth (xerostomia)

Because of the prevalence of medications being taken in this age range, for conditions ranging from diabetes to blood pressure to cancer treatment, dry mouth is a common occurrence. Not only does this usually result in bad breath, but the lack of the mouth's natural

---

37   Claudia Hammond, "Is age the cause of receding gums?" BBC Future, last modified August 7, 2013, http://www.bbc.com/future/story/20130807-does-age-damage-your-gums

cleanser—saliva—means that cavities are starting to come back into play, and habits to combat the condition, such as sucking on sugary cough drops or hard candies, aren't helping the situation.

Dry mouth can also be a problem for denture wearers, as the lack of saliva can make the dentures feel loose in the mouth, leading to discomfort. In these cases, a denture fixative and/or artificial saliva can help, as can drinking sips of water frequently throughout the day. Other options for combating dry mouth include:

- Chewing sugarless gum

- Sucking on sugarless candies

- Avoiding alcohol or caffeinated beverages

- Avoiding tobacco

Varnish for a Healthier Smile

Even though cavities may seem like something only kids have to worry about, the fact is that the rate of tooth decay for people ages sixty-five-plus is now exceeding the rate of cavities in schoolchildren.[38] Part of this is due to those two age-related conditions mentioned earlier: dry mouth and gum recession. As the lack of self-cleaning saliva becomes more prevalent and more of that soft root tissue becomes exposed, the risk of developing cavities increases, particularly along the gum line.

To get ahead of that risk, more dentists are beginning to recommend a fluoride varnish around the base, or neck, of the teeth. The varnish, which usually consists of anywhere between .1 percent

---

38   "The aging mouth – and how to keep it younger," Harvard Health
      Publishing, Harvard Medical School, last modified January 2010,
      https://www.health.harvard.edu/diseases-and-conditions/
      the-aging-mouth-and-how-to-keep-it-younger

and 5 percent sodium fluoride and a resin or synthetic base that helps it stick to the teeth, sets rapidly and can be applied quickly, reducing the time that the hygienist spends in the mouth and minimizing the risk of gagging or accidental swallowing of the product.

While the majority of studies into the effectiveness of fluoride varnishes in preventing cavities have been conducted on children, more researchers are beginning to look into its impact on older adults. For children, systematic reviews have proven how effective topical fluoride can be in preventing or slowing the progress of cavities. With older adults, recent reviews have also shown a reduction in root cavities, with fluoride varnish controlling root cavities better than brushing with a high fluoride toothpaste alone. The study concluded that fluoride varnishes on older adults, particularly those who have difficulty brushing, would benefit from varnish being applied to the base of the teeth three to four times a year.[39]

Dental Implants and Dentures

More and more, implants are becoming the norm over dentures when it comes to replacing missing teeth. There are multiple reasons why— the main one being that implants look and act like real teeth. This doesn't just mean being able to tear into a corn-on-the-cob anytime you want—it also applies to how the implant acts in the mouth.

With dentures, the offending teeth are removed from the mouth and nothing replaces them. Over time, the body reabsorbs the bone that the teeth were removed from since it's no longer supporting teeth, leading to the degradation and thinning of the jaw. Implants,

---

39   Nicola Innes and Dafydd Evans, "Caries prevention for older people in residential care homes," *Evidence-Based Dentistry* 10, no. 3 (2009): 83–87, https://doi. org/10.1038/sj.ebd.6400672

however, are made with a material that bonds with the bone, acting like real teeth so that the body isn't stimulated to begin reabsorption.

Other benefits include comfort—implants act like real teeth instead of shifting in the mouth or requiring fixatives, as dentures do—and longevity. The typical implant has a failure rate of less than 5 percent and lasts an average of twenty-five years, with some said to last a lifetime. Meanwhile, the lifecycle of dentures is usually anywhere from seven to fifteen years.[40]

Implants are also a healthier option for the surrounding teeth, as well. When a bridge is placed, for instance, the two teeth adjacent to the area need to be ground down so that they can hold the bridge structure. Consequently, these newly worn teeth are more vulnerable to decay and damage.

How are Implants Implanted?

The implant procedure typically involves placing a titanium screw in just the right place in the jawbone, followed by the attachment of the prosthetic tooth. In some cases, patients may opt for a combination of implant and denture, in which a series of titanium screws are implanted in the jaw, with the external end shaped so that a partial or full denture can be snapped onto it.

Implants don't work for all patients, however. If you smoke, have diabetes, or have substantial bone loss already, implants may not be the best option.

---

40   Lesley Alderman, "For Most, Implants Beat Dentures, but at a Price," Health, The New York Times, last modified July 30, 2010, http://www.nytimes.com/2010/07/31/health/31patient.html

What to Know Before Whitening Older Teeth

As the outer layer of enamel thins, the dentin underneath becomes more visible, making teeth appear less white. Coffee, red wine, tea, and tobacco can also stain teeth, leading them to potentially look older than they are.

While over-the-counter whitening products and whitening toothpastes can help lighten teeth by a few shades, the effects are often much less dramatic in older teeth. However, before going through with a full-on dental whitening, keep in mind that professional whitening procedures may leave teeth feeling more sensitive and some stains may be more challenging to remove than others, requiring several rounds of bleaching before they can be removed.

Are Teeth Affected by Osteoporosis?

Osteoporosis, a medical condition that decreases the density of bones and makes them more likely to fracture, can also affect the bone density in the mouth. According to a study by the National Institute of Health, women with osteoporosis were three times more likely to have a loose tooth than women without the condition.[41]

Watching Out for Signs of Oral Cancer

As is the case with most cancers, the risk of oral cancer increases with age and the use of tobacco products. With each year that someone smokes or chews tobacco, the risk of developing oral cancer increases.

When oral cancer does develop, it's most likely to develop on the lower lip first, followed by the upper lip and then the tongue. Initial

---

41 "Oral Health and Bone Disease," NIH Osteoporosis and Related Bone Diseases National Resource Center, https://www.bones.nih.gov/health-info/bone/bone-health/oral-health/oral-health-and-bone-disease

signs and symptoms of the disease are easy to miss, but if you notice a white or red patch on your lip, tongue, or bottom of your mouth that lasts longer than two weeks, let your dentist know about it. While it may be the early signs of oral cancer, there's also the chance that it could be a sore caused by herpes or yeast infection, which, while painful, can also be treated.

Dental Care and Dementia

Older adults suffering from forms of dementia such as Alzheimer's disease should be allowed to conduct their own dental care for as long as they can, with reminders from family and caregivers, and supervision if needed. Establishing a daily care routine in the early stages of dementia is particularly important as assistance in brushing teeth may be needed later on.

Since it can often be challenging to communicate with someone who has dementia, it may be hard to tell if that person is suffering from mouth pain or discomfort. If you're a caregiver or family member of someone with dementia, it can help to keep an eye out for the following signs of potential dental problems:

- Refusing to eat hot or cold foods, or any food

- Frequent pulling at the face and mouth

- Increased moaning, shouting, or restlessness

- Refusal to take part in daily activities

- Aggressive behavior

- Disturbed sleep

- Not wearing dentures[42]

---

42   "Dental Care," Alzheimer's Society, https://www.alzheimers.org.uk/info/20029/daily_living/9/dental_care/3

Dental Treatment for those Suffering from Dementia

According to the Alzheimer's Society, dental treatment for those suffering from dementia should be considered with all of the stages of dementia in mind. During the early stages, for instance, dentists should recommend and conduct treatment with the understanding that the patient will not be able to care for his or her own teeth at some point. Therefore, preventative treatments for conditions such as gum disease are very important. As the disease progresses, patients may need sedation or general anesthesia for dental visits, and their ability to cooperate during these visits should be assessed beforehand. In the late stages of dementia, the challenges of thinking clearly along with physical frailty and often additional complex medical conditions can make dental visits challenging, and care should mainly focus on maintaining the patient's comfort, preventing dental disease, and providing emergency treatment.[43]

When considering dental treatment for dementia patients, the following factors should be kept in mind:

- What dental problems are being experienced

- Whether the patient is able to give informed consent

- The patient's level of independence, thinking abilities, physical impairments, cooperation and mental state.

Once these conditions are assessed, the dentist can provide input on the best treatment options for the patient, and how regularly he or she should see the dentist.

As with every stage of life, keeping teeth in their best condition requires regular maintenance and common sense practices. With this

---

43   Ibid.

in mind, a little effort now can make a big difference in the teeth you get to keep—and their overall health—down the road.

Conclusion

I hope you enjoyed reading this book as much as I enjoyed writing it! I hope you have found it helpful in what to look for regarding your oral health care.

As with the beginning chapter of this book being about my life story, there are many important people who are also an integral part of this continuing journey. The most important being my wife Jenny, who I have been married to, at the time this book was written, almost seventeen years! She has been my rock and I truly would not be where I am without her and what she does to make me a better person, husband, father, and dentist.

My children Rachel and Connor, who have had to go sometimes without a dad who was working and helping other people have been

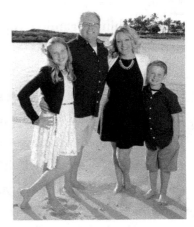

Dr. Benson and his family.

very understanding and have had fun watching and learning about business. Their understanding of the greater calling cannot be understated and that makes them amazing kids!

Other extended family I would like to thank are my in-laws, Pat and Sheila Talbot, who have also seen me grow and supported our family tremendously along the way.

I have been blessed with some amazing colleagues and specialist to work with. Dr. Ralph Reynolds, an extremely talented oral surgeon, has taught be a great deal about quality surgical care and he was the first person to greet me when I first arrived in Greeley. It has been a privilege to work with him and I look forward to many more years! Dr. David Richter, in my opinion the best orthodontist in Greeley and possibly northern Colorado, has been one of my closest friends, and we have successfully treated many cases and changed several lives through our treatment goals and charitable work.

And last, but certainly not least, is the Catholic Church, who through God's grace I have been given this amazing gift of life and passion for dentistry.

People sometimes forget the dentist until they have pain and usually by then, it is too late to avoid a more invasive procedure. As with anything regarding your health, prevention is key. And with dentistry today, we have the ability, materials, and technology to make prevention more accessible than it has ever been.

Winston Churchill once said, "We make a living by what we get, but we make a life by what we give." And I live by that statement—I'm not satisfied with my work until my patients have a healthy smile that gives them back their confidence and happiness. And you shouldn't be satisfied with your smile until yours brings you that same joy.

For more information, or if you'd like to book an appointment, please call us at (970) 281-5972, contact us by email at DrBuddy@ida-greeley.com, or visit our website at www.ida-greeley.com.

CPSIA information can be obtained
at www.ICGtesting.com
Printed in the USA
FSHW022040090419
57116FS